Culture, Ethics, and Advance Care Planning

Culture, Ethics, and Advance Care Planning

Alissa Hurwitz Swota

LEXINGTON BOOKS
A division of

ROWMAN & LITTLEFIELD PUBLISHERS, INC.
Lanham • Boulder • New York • Toronto • Plymouth, UK

Published by Lexington Books
A division of Rowman & Littlefield Publishers, Inc.
A wholly owned subsidiary of The Rowman & Littlefield Publishing Group, Inc.
4501 Forbes Boulevard, Suite 200, Lanham, Maryland 20706
http://www.lexingtonbooks.com

Estover Road, Plymouth PL6 7PY, United Kingdom

British Library Cataloguing in Publication Information Available

Library of Congress Cataloging-in-Publication Data

Swota, Alissa Hurwitz.
   Culture, ethics, and advance care planning / Alissa Hurwitz Swota.
      p. ; cm.
   Includes bibliographical references and index.
   ISBN 978-0-7391-3565-5 (cloth : alk. paper)
   ISBN 978-0-7391-3567-9 (electronic)
   1. Advance directives (Medical care) 2. Transcultural medical care. I. Title.
   [DNLM: 1. Advance Care Planning--ethics. 2. Cultural Competency. 3. Cultural
Diversity. 4. Professional-Patient Relations. W 85.5. S979c 2009]
   R726.2.S96 2009
   362.1--dc22   2009020293

Printed in the United States of America

∞™ The paper used in this publication meets the minimum requirements of American
National Standard for Information Sciences—Permanence of Paper for Printed Library
Materials, ANSI/NISO Z39.48-1992.

Printed in the United States of America

To Joel and Hannah, with love

Contents

Acknowledgments

I would not have been able to write this book if not for the help of numerous people. The idea to even write a book and the helpful "nudge" to develop a proposal is due to my mentor, advisor, sounding board, and above all, friend, Bonnie Steinbock. She has looked over my work since I was her graduate student and her meticulous and careful comments have always proven to be invaluable. To her I owe a debt of gratitude that I can only hope to begin to repay. Another person who has helped with this book from the proposal stage is Ken Goodman. Without his help this book truly would not have been possible. His insights are consistently brilliant and his patience is unparalleled. He afforded me vast amounts of time and advice, and for that I thank him. Another person responsible for getting this book off the ground is Mark Kuczewski. He helped me swim through publishing questions and gave so much of his time and patience to what were often sophomoric questions. He was always available for guidance and thoughtful comments. His wisdom and kindness are only a few of his admirable traits and I cannot thank him enough for all of his support.

I would also like to thank all of the people that I worked with during my postdoctoral fellowship at the University of Toronto Joint Centre for Bioethics. During my time at the Joint Centre I was exposed to so many of the issues that I write about in the book. Even more, I was privileged enough to work with leaders in the field of clinical bioethics, whose wisdom ran both deep and broad. I was particularly fortunate to get to work with Kerry Bowman, an expert in cultural issues in bioethics. Kerry is a spectacular teacher, scholar, and friend. He allowed me to bounce ideas off of him from the infancy of this book. He always had some profound advice and new twist on the issues. To him, I owe a special thank you.

While writing this book I received a research grant from the University of North Florida. This grant allowed me an entire summer to focus my efforts on writing. Affording young faculty with such a luxury is a gift and for that I thank the people at The University of North Florida. I have also received support from the Blue Cross Blue Shield of Northeast Florida Center for Ethics, Public Policy, and the Professions at the University of North Florida, at which I am a fellow. I want to thank A. David Kline, the director of the Center, for all of his help throughout the writing process. I also want to thank my colleagues in the Department of Philosophy at The University of North Florida for all of their patience and advice. In addition, I would be remiss if I did not thank the research assistants, Andrew Sun, Amber Hines, and especially, Colleen Gatliff who helped me with everything from gathering sources to formatting my bibliography. All of them made my road a bit less arduous.

The people at Lexington Books have been extremely helpful and it has been my pleasure and good fortune to be able to work with them. I would especially like to thank my editor, Julie Kirsch. She was always available with a quick response to my questions and offered wonderful advice.

Thanks also to my mother, Gail Hurwitz, for a lifetime of support. Most of all, I would like to thank my husband, Joel. He listened to ideas without hesitation and was generous in offering his priceless insights. He pointed out the end when I was sure that there was none in sight. He watched our daughter, Hannah, so that I could get a few more hours out of the days. He is my rock, my best friend, and one of the people to whom the book is dedicated. I am sure that it is largely because of his love and support that this book was possible.

Introduction

It is more important to know what sort of a patient has a disease, than what sort of disease a patient has.

—Sir William Osler, 1911

Any care that fails to include cultural considerations falls short of the human needs that must be met

—Loustanna and Sobo, 1997

From its inception, biomedicine[1] has endorsed the principle of autonomy, often considering it to override other competing values at play in the clinical setting. The automatic deference to physician authority ended by the 1970s. Prior to that time, the ruling dictum was "doctor knows best." Paternalism reigned supreme and patient autonomy consisted in choosing meals from the hospital menu. With the advent of bioethics, the pendulum moved from physician paternalism to patient autonomy, at least in the United States.[2] The voice of the patient gained an important place in the medical decision-making process, with patient values taking on a leading role. To be sure, at the turn of the twenty-first century, skepticism about the absolute authority of autonomy began to be voiced.[3] Nevertheless, in the clinical setting, such skepticism has been rare.

The emphasis on patient autonomy, and respect for the values and preferences of patients, has extended beyond competent patients to previously competent patients, whose prior wishes are often deemed decisive for making treatment decisions. Advance directives enable individuals to retain control over their medical fates even after they are no longer competent to express

1

their values and preferences. This is most important when there is a discrepancy between the values of the patient and the views of treating physicians about what is medically indicated. Until relatively recently, when patient preferences clashed with "medical indications," it was not even perceived as a genuine conflict between legitimate interests: conventional medical practice usually prevailed. Today, patient preferences have gained a highly influential role in the medical decision-making process. Indeed, when patient preferences conflict with medical indications, the former receive top billing in terms of priority.[4]

For the most part, biomedicine has regarded the pride of place given to autonomy as a triumph. It lauds those who "take the initiative" and make plans for what is to be done in case of future illness and possible incompetence The importance of autonomy is reflected in advance care planning, a process through which an individual makes known her preferences concerning medical treatment, in case she becomes incompetent, by, for example, drafting a living will or by appointing another individual—usually called a health care proxy—to make decisions for her.[5] Advance care planning is a way of ensuring that the patient's wishes are carried out, and thus promoting patient autonomy. It is also a way of relieving family members of the burden of determining what the patient "would have wanted," when he or she is no longer capable of expressing preference. Reinforcing this "relief" role of directives, one study reported that 70 percent of patients had a positive attitude toward advance directives, due in part to "their ability to help preserve autonomy and relieve relatives of the 'burden' of making difficult decisions" (Stephens as cited in Berry and Singer 1998, 1571).

With front page stories like the Florida case of Terry Schiavo, as well as the older cases of Karen Ann Quinlan and Nancy Cruzan, advance care planning in general and advance directives in particular were thrust into the spotlight and became concepts familiar to a large audience. As one commentator on the Cruzan case noted, "If Nancy Cruzan had had an advance directive, her care could have been terminated six and one-half years before it was actually terminated. . . . With an advance directive Nancy Cruzan could have died without a court battle in most states" (Ulrich 1999, 36). By highlighting the negative side of medical technology in which the quantity of life is extended while the quality is markedly decreased, these cases served as a wake-up call. Through their suffering, all of those involved in these headline cases made it clear that medical technology is unbelievably powerful and that we ought to have a healthy respect for it. We must be aware of the consequences of utilizing it and let others know of our preferences regarding it. At the very least, these cases highlighted the utility of making such preferences known (e.g., through advance directives) by giving a face to the suffering that may have been avoided had some difficult conversations taken place and such documents been drafted. As advance directives gained residence in the public consciousness, the hope was that discussions concerning what one would want done in case of incompetence, which conditions are acceptable and which are not, and which values ought to guide the decision-making process for medical treatments, would occur with greater frequency. These conversations needed to take place. Whether they occurred over the breakfast table or during large family gatherings like Thanksgiving dinner, with the whole family present, they just needed to take place.

This imperative—to be an active participant in planning for one's own future medical treatment—is founded on the presupposition that all people value open discussion about illness and medical decision making. Legislation has supported this presupposition in the United States and clinical medicine has adopted this practice. However, this "one size fits all" approach to planning for health care in advance and communicating about illness[6] in general does not reflect an accurate picture of a society in which one finds a plurality of cultures. For instance, while engaging in planning for future illness is viewed by some as a way of making sure that authorship of the last chapter of life is undertaken by the person whose life narrative is being penned, for others, it is a violation of their values. Questions about treatment preferences in the face of life-threatening illness might be construed as cruel, offensive, arrogant, rude, or even an invitation for disease. Seen in this way, advance directives, despite their original intent, are viewed as having the potential to harm (Werth et al. 2002, 207–8). To be sure, what constitutes "harm" can vary widely. What is seen as a beneficial endeavor to some—engaging in discussions about future medical treatment—may be seen by others as an attack on one's belief system. As Marshall et al. found in their survey of Navajo patients, health providers, and traditional healers, "86 percent of the individuals interviewed considered discussion of advance care planning for near-death medical decisions a dangerous violation of Navajo values" (Marshall et al., as cited in Swota 2008, 121). The following case does well to illustrate the complications that can arise when engaging in advance care planning in a culturally diverse setting:

Mr. Carho is a 76 year old Navajo man who presents with complaints of fatigue, dizziness, and general malaise. He also informs his doctor that he has recently started to forget even the simplest of things. He enters a room and forgets what he was looking for. On several occasions he has had problems with his speech, has forgotten basic words, and the names of various family members. Mr. Carho has also begun to exhibit impaired motor and spatial skills. He lives with his wife of 25 years. Until now, both he and his wife have been relatively healthy. After running an extensive series of tests based on Mr. Carho's medical history and symptoms, his doctor determines that Mr. Carho is showing symptoms of early dementia. In addition to explaining his findings and various ways of coping with the symptoms mentioned above, Mr. Carho's physician, who has been caring for Mr. Carho for several years, decides that now would be a good time to bring up advance directives and start the process of advance care planning. Such planning seemed extremely appropriate in light of the new diagnosis. Soon after attempting to open a dialogue on advance care planning, beginning with an explanation of what such planning entails, Mr. Carho and his wife become visibly shaken and plead with the physician to stop discussing such matters. Confused and worried that she has upset her patient, Mr. Carho's physician reiterates the plan of care and leaves the room. Still unclear as to what happened, she starts to question why such a "good thing"—bringing up advance care planning with a long-time patient—could have ended so badly.

To be sure, Mr. Carho's physician had the best of intentions—to elucidate her patient's values and preferences concerning medical treatment in case he became unable to express such wishes on his own. She thought that given his current diagnosis of a disease with identifiable and foreseeable consequences, they could make plans for potential future incompetence with great insight and awareness. Mr. Carho would have a very privileged, informed perspective from which to make decisions about medical treatment in the future. How great it would be to take the burden off loved ones who, with Mr. Carho's preferences and values out in the open, would in turn be able to make more informed decisions.

From the Carho's perspective, what the physician did was far from a thoughtful act that might serve them well in the future. Rather, it was an insolent act at best, and at worst, potentially harmful.[7] Briefly, it was disrespectful because, "In Navajo culture, an important concept is 'Hozho' that involves goodness, harmony, positive attitude, and universal beauty. Negative thoughts of illness raised in discussions of advance health planning conflict with this philosophy" (Berger as cited in Swota 2008, 122). A belief in the Navajo culture is that control of events such as death lies not with the individual, but rather, is determined by fate. To think that individuals can control something as great as death is foolish.

Cases like this will only become more common as the demographics in societies reflect increasingly diverse populations. In order for advance care planning to flourish, for it to be able to achieve the goal of providing individuals with a way to maintain control over their "post-competent" fate[8] while at the same time not offending or harming some members of society, it is necessary to determine how to approach advance care planning in a culturally sensitive manner. Professional groups such as The American Academy of Family Physicians (AAFP) have joined in the call for greater awareness of the influence culture has on the medical encounter. The AAFP has engaged in a threefold effort to increase cultural awareness and sensitivity, publishing cultural proficiency guidelines and policy, along with advocacy statements in their educational activities (Searight et al. 2005, 515). Principle 5 in the AAFP's policy statement on end-of-life care states that "Care at the end of life should recognize, assess, and address the psychological, social, spiritual/religious issues, and cultural taboos realizing that different cultures may require significantly different approaches" (Searight et al. 2005, 515). Support for achieving greater cultural sensitivity[9] and awareness, in order to be successful, needs to be buttressed by methods and tools with which such ends can be achieved.

This issue of attaining greater cultural sensitivity in advance care planning underscores the more general need to focus greater attention on the "cultural conflicts" that arise in the clinical setting. For too long, there has been an assumption in clinical ethics in particular and bioethics in general, that there is a "common morality (to greater and lesser extent)," and a failure to recognize "The possibility of 'incommensurable' moral languages, 'deep' rifts in moral understandings, and a plurality of conflicting moral norms" (Turner HCA 2003, 113). Galanti describes this same idea by noting that, "No matter how much 'evidence' is presented to the contrary, people rarely change or even question their worldviews. Instead, they reinterpret events in a manner consistent with their beliefs" (Galanti 2003, 10). In this book I want to acknowledge such differences and the frustrations born from the fractured starting point at which clinical encounters often begin—a place where values conflict and concepts and frameworks may vary widely.[10] Put another way, current demographic trends "suggest that at least one of every four patients [seen] in the clinical setting will not share [the] cultural, ethnic, or linguistic heritage" of their physician (Kukoyi 2005, 389). There might not be anything akin to advance care planning in some cultures, in others, the idea of looking toward the future makes no sense, and still in others, engaging in conversations about potential dire prognoses and terminal conditions (conversations common to advance care planning) is tantamount to inviting great harms to befall an individual. My hope is to provide a guide that focuses on navigating the difficult terrain of advance care planning in a diverse, pluralistic clinical setting. In short, in our struggle to gain control over the medical decision-making process, ending ultimately in the "triumph of autonomy," we lost sight of the fact that not everyone had joined in the fight.

The idea of allowing individuals to retain some control in shaping their futures, even when that future includes incompetence, permeates not only the prized values of biomedicine, but also, in the United States, occupies a spot in federal legislation.[11] And, while legislation provides a practical driving force behind becoming increasingly more culturally sensitive, I maintain that becoming culturally sensitive is an essential component of providing quality health care. Specifically, health care providers[12] "must continue the struggle to communicate complex and often frightening information across barriers of language and culture. [Health care providers] who dismiss the need for communication skills and a culturally sensitive approach to making medical decisions do so at the risk of providing substandard care"[13] (Powell as cited in Swota 2008, 110).

Broaching the topic of advance care planning is mandated in our society. Such planning is contrary to the practices of some cultures. As such, something must be done in order to decrease the likelihood of conflict posed by the current conditions. In order for advance care planning to make sense to individuals from various cultures and to decrease the likelihood of deeply offending individuals from others, advance care planning must be situated within a multicultural context. Given how entrenched advance care planning is in the medical context, to not attempt to engage in the process in a culturally sensitive way smacks of a dangerous indifference. Some good advice is to remember, "No one individual can anticipate all the problems that might arise in an attempt to understand chronic illness and disability in a multicultural society, but we can all have enough sensitivity to realize that there might be significant differences, and enough respect for others to ask questions and listen carefully to the replies" (Groce and Zola as cited in Loustaunau and Sobo 1997, 146). It is my hope that this book will provide much-needed guidance in a scantily charted territory. Ultimately this book should serve as a resource in helping individuals grapple with the issues born at the intersection of clashing cultures and advance care planning, and serve as a guide for advance care planning in a multicultural society.

Roadmap

The first section of the book will include an overview of the foundations of advance care planning—what it is, why it is important, what function it serves in health care, and some of the criticisms it has faced. Such a discussion is necessary not only in order to gain an understanding of advance directives and the advance care planning process, but also, to become aware of the criticisms waged against it even within a system in which autonomy is a highly prized value. This awareness will help one to appreciate the issues that come up when dealing with advance directives and advance care planning across cultures. Also included in this first section is a brief look at some of the legislation, both in the United States and abroad, concerning advance care planning. Next, I will analyze the concept of cultural sensitivity, making clear that an essential element of being a good health care provider is being culturally sensitive. I will use cases to identify and elucidate various issues that may arise in a culturally diverse clinical setting. Finally, I will focus on specific tools and frameworks that have been developed to help health care providers practice in a multicultural setting. I will look at tools that will help to facilitate cross-cultural communication in health care in general, and others that will help providers engage specifically in advance care planning in a culturally sensitive manner. Culturally sensitive providers are limited, to some extent, by the organizational mandates and professional tenets which inform their practices and set the boundaries within which they provide care. As such, I will look at cultural sensitivity at the organizational level and in terms of what various professional bodies have called for in an effort to increase cultural sensitivity in healthcare.

In examining these issues, I will be employing generalizations about different cultural groups.[14] However, this should not be taken to imply that one can determine the views of others based solely on things such as last name or place of birth. Rather, I want to point out that there are a number of issues involved in medical decision making in general and advance care planning in particular—issues on which one can find a wide variation of views driven by values that are prioritized in vastly different ways. I will use generalizations as a heuristic device, a way to make manifest some of the different perspectives people may take on the deeply personal issues so central to advance care planning. By no means are these generalizations meant to imply that cultures are monolithic. Generalizations can help health care providers generate hypotheses "about particular cultural beliefs, values, and practices . . . but then [the health care provider] must assess the degree to which an individual patient or family might adhere to their cultural background, if at all" (Kawaga-Singer and Kassim-Lakha 2003, 582). Galanti draws a nice distinction between a generalization and a stereotype:

> The difference between a stereotype and a generalization lies not in the *content*, but in the *usage* of the information. . . . A stereotype is an ending point. No attempt is made to learn whether the individual fits the statement. . . . A generalization, on the other hand, is a beginning point. It indicates common trends, but further information is needed to ascertain whether the statement is appropriate to a particular individual"(Galanti 2003, 4).

Thus, while generalizations are useful insofar as they may serve to make health care providers aware of the diversity of beliefs and practices they may encounter in the clinical setting, it is paramount that providers recognize that each patient must be viewed as an individual to whom generalizations may be more or less applicable. Attempting to gain any substantive insight by building on a foundation of stereotypes would be an effort made in vain. As Wright et al. explain "there is no typical family. With respect to culture, each family

is unique in composition, decision-making style, and degree of acculturation"
(Wright et al. 1997, 66).

The clinical reality is one in which diversity abounds, time is a scarce resource, and matters of the utmost importance are being decided and negotiated
amongst strangers who often bring to the encounter disparate worldviews.
Given this setting, the only assumptions that should be made are that assumptions are dangerous, that stereotypes can wreak havoc in the clinical setting, and
that good communication needs to take into account the reality of diversity in
the clinical context. Koenig and Gates-Williams do well to summarize an ideal
approach to patient care against a backdrop of multiculturalism:

> the challenge of respecting diversity is great. Because culture is fluid and
> dynamic, how can we respect differences while avoiding stereotyping of
> patients? The answer is clear. Patients should never be approached as empty
> vessels, as bearers of particular cultures. Rather, it is essential to approach
> patients first as unique persons, assessing them within the context of their
> family or other key social support system. General knowledge about theo-
> retical groups is helpful. . . . Nonetheless, clinical inferences about cultural
> differences must be evaluated for relevance to a particular patient or family.
> (Koenig and Gates-Williams 1995, 247)

Primarily, I want to raise awareness regarding the diversity of views and
guiding norms that people have regarding health and illness more generally
and in particular, in relation to the issues raised in the advance care planning
process. While this book will not, indeed cannot provide an algorithm, a way
of approaching *every* case and ensuring that no cultural conflicts will develop,
it will provide needed guidance on how to avert and defuse the charged encounters that may occur when cultures clash in the clinical setting.

NOTES

1. I have chosen to use the term "biomedicine" to refer to a system of medicine
that "originates from within the perspective of European and American scientifi-
cally based medicine," it is "generally referred to as the benchmark medical system"
(Loustanna and Sobo 1997, 3). To be sure, there are several other terms that could be
used (e.g., Western medicine), but I will be consistent in employing this term throughout the text. In addition, I will be focusing on biomedicine as it is experienced within
the clinical setting. That is, while bioethicists have criticized the idea of autonomy
uber alles, *in the clinical setting*, there has not been the same skepticism (Bonnie
Steinbock, personal correspondence July 1, 2008).

2. In other countries, physician paternalism has remained dominant (e.g., in Italy;
see Ripamonti 1999).

3. See Gaylin and Jennings 2003, as well as O'Neill 2002.

4. The classic case of the priority given to patient preferences, even in the face of a medical treatment that can offer "complete cure," is that of a Jehovah's Witness refusing a blood transfusion. Thus, even in cases where a transfusion would result in a complete reversal of the ailment at issue, the values of the patient—here not to accept any blood or blood products—trump. In addition, it is not uncommon in the clinical setting to see the treatment recommendations of health care practitioners passed over in favor of alternatives that align more readily with preferences of patients and families. To be sure, this is even the case when the treatment recommendations of medical professionals offer a much higher likelihood of success (e.g., in terms of relieving pain and curing disease). For the most part, there is an emphasis on shared decision making. Interestingly, studies have shown that patients need to see more benefit from a proposed treatment before accepting it than a physician would (see Montgomery and Fahey 2001).

5. I will describe advance care planning and advance directives in much greater detail in chapters 1 and 2.

6. I will understand the concept of illness, in contrast to disease, in the following way, "Whereas disease defines a pathophysiologic process, illness is defined by the complete person—physical, psychological, social, and cultural. Illness represents an individual's unique and personal experience of being unwell" (Green et al. 2002, 142). Kleinman et al. explain the distinction between disease and illness as follows, "disease in the Western medical paradigm is malfunctioning or maladaptation of biologic and psychophysiologic processes in the individual; whereas illness represents personal, interpersonal, and cultural reactions to disease or discomfort. . . . Because illness experience is an intimate part of social systems of meaning and rules for behavior, it is strongly influenced by culture: it is . . . culturally constructed" (Kleinman et al. 1978, 252).

7. For a nice discussion of the principle of respect for autonomy and how it might translate into the Navajo culture, see Taylor 2004.

8. This term comes from Norman Cantor; see Cantor 1992.

9. While many use the term "cultural competence," I will be using the term "cultural sensitivity" throughout this book. As one cultural competency manager explains,

"A lot of people in the field have never been comfortable with the term cultural competence." "One never really becomes 100 percent competent in this evolving field. We're not trying to imply that you can become competent." Cultural sensitivity, cross-cultural practice, cultural pluralism, patient-centered care—all of these terms are being used to describe the same basic goal of eliminating the barriers to health care that are caused by cultural differences. (Butterfield, www.acponline.org/clinical_information/journals_publications/acp_hospitalist/mar08/cover.htm#sb1, accessed July 17, 2008)

10. The differences at issue run so deep and are so fundamental, that the concept of an advance directive is not even able to be translated with ease into some languages: "the concept of advance directives . . . is not easily translated into the Korean language" (Ersek et al. 1998, 1688).

11. Here I am referring to the Patient Self-Determination Act, which I will examine in more depth in chapter 1.

12. I will adopt a broad conception of "health care provider" for the rest of the book. Specifically, it is not only bedside caregivers that are included in this group, but also administrators and policy makers, among others, who are responsible for the direction of care provided at a particular health care institution.

13. Bracketed sections are my emendation.

14. I do not maintain that cultures are monolithic, nor do I hold that the effect that one's culture has on how the world is viewed is something that is easily delineated. As Turner explains,

> most scholars acknowledge that life experiences, level of education, socioeconomic status, family history and degree of acculturation render meaningless monolithic, unitary, all-encompassing characterizations of seamless "cultures," heuristic tools such as the concepts of "local moral worlds" and "horizons of meaning" play a meaningful explanatory role in delineating variations in modes of moral reasoning. (Turner 2003, 108–9)

I will focus on the role of culture in determining "modes of moral reasoning" in advance care planning.

Chapter One

Advance Care Planning:
A Focus on Process

I will not allow a specialist to decide when to let me go. I will choose my own way, or at least make the elements of my own way so clear, that the choice, should I be unable, can be made by those who know me best.

—Sherwin Nuland, 1994

Tell me how you die and I will tell you who you are.

—Mexican Folk Saying
(as cited in DeSpelder and Strickland 2001)

Prior to discussing the issues that surround advance care planning in a multicultural setting, one needs to understand the driving forces behind the evolution of advance care planning in the biomedical model, and appreciate what it is that many find appealing about advance directives and advance care planning in the first place. Why are advance directives and advance care planning so entrenched in many Western societies? How have they built up so much currency? In exploring these questions and answers offered to them, one can begin to gain a better understanding of why advance directives have garnered so much attention and what it is that they represent in the biomedical model. To be sure, their status in the biomedical model aligns readily with an individualistic conception of the self that reveres autonomy. Such an idea, while foundational to the biomedical model,[1] is one that might bewilder those from cultures in which individuals are understood only within a broader context of a family or group, and facilitating the exercise of patient autonomy is not paramount.

The pace of medical technology is rapid. Born from the advances in technology are countless benefits. Diagnosing illness in the earliest of stages, performing intricate surgeries in utero, and procuring organs from one person and implanting them in another—these are no longer possibilities, but rather par for the clinical course. These advances underscore the proficiency we have developed at keeping people alive longer, staving off death even in what seem to be the gravest of circumstances. Staying the hand of death is pursued with a zealousness that is premised, at least in part, on the notion that death is always and inherently bad—something over which we need to gain control and avoid for as long as possible.

It is no surprise that individuals might want control over how they die. Control is something that we have gained over so many other aspects of our lives, why not over medical care and what the end of life will look like? Entrenched in U.S. law, this idea was expressed eloquently by Justice Cardoza in *Schloendorff* (1914) when he maintained that, "Every adult human being of adult years and sound mind has a right to determine what shall be done with his own body." Even more, "a surgeon who performs an operation without his patient's consent commits an assault, for which he is liable in damages." *Schloendorff*[2] represents a milestone insofar as it identifies an obligation on the part of health care professionals to include patient preferences in the medical decision-making process. Not only is an obligation demarcated, there are teeth behind it as well in the form of "damages" to be provided if the obligation is not met. This decision paved the way for informed consent to gain residence as a mainstay in the clinical context. To be sure, such residency was a result of a hard-fought battle for patient control and autonomy in the medical decision-making process.[3] Autonomy stands as the driving principle behind informed consent requirements that aim to "give power to patients who have traditionally not spoken and have been powerless in light of medical proficiency and authority" (Kettle 2003, 43). Briefly, criteria necessary for a patient to give informed consent[4] are adequate information, voluntariness, and capacity. That is, the patient must be provided with relevant information, be able to understand and process this information, and come to a decision without undue influences. Informed consent requirements stand as a means by which the autonomy of competent patients is recognized and cultivated.

It stands to reason that if one has dedicated a lifetime to developing a certain sort of life story or narrative, to take away authorship right before the final chapter is penned is unfair at best and at worst a deep harm to the individual. To deny an individual control over such an important issue seems to fly in the face of our nature as rational agents, capable of complex thought and action. As Norman Cantor explains,

Having a hand in determining how you live your last days is a critical component in an individual's ability to follow her conception of a good life and the

values and interests involved in such a life till the very end. Being left without a
voice, forced to let others decide what is best seems to run contrary to the ideal
of self-determination. (Cantor 1993, 30)

Control in such cases translates into having a means by which one can
maintain control over her life, even after incompetence. One important way
to maintain such control is through the process of advance care planning.
Advance care planning has been heralded as "highly relevant to the quality of health care" and a process that "helps optimize beneficial treatment
decisions" (Pearlman et al. 1995, 354). Advance care planning is a process
in which individuals discuss and elucidate their values and preferences with
regard to medical treatment, in case of a future time in which they are inca-
pable of participating in such decisions. Engaging in such discussions provides the patient with an opportunity to clarify values and principles that are
fundamental to her life story, providing health care professionals with a much
deeper understanding of the patient as a person. To be sure, the information
obtained through a thoughtful advance care planning process can also be useful in provider-patient relationships while the patient is still competent. During the advance care planning process, individuals might specify in writing
which types of treatments they would and would not prefer, conditions under
which such preferences obtain, and specific values that ought to guide the
development of the medical treatment plan. The resulting document is a form
of advance directive known as a "living will." A living will typically delin-
eates the patient's preferences for medical treatments, providing guidance to
health care providers and family members when the patient is no longer able
to convey such preferences for herself.

Another form of advance directive that might evolve out of the advance care
planning process is a durable power of attorney for health care or health care
proxy. These advance directives designate an individual or individuals to speak
for the patient in case the patient is not able to do so for herself. The appointed
individuals are called "surrogates" or "proxies" depending upon jurisdiction.[5]
Surrogates must be both willing and able to make decisions on behalf of the
incompetent patient. Decisions are to be based on the substituted judgment
standard. According to this standard, surrogates, based on their knowledge of
the patient, must ask themselves what the patient would have wanted if she
was able to make a decision based on the current circumstances. Where no
such knowledge of the patient exists, surrogates are to make a decision based
on the patient's best interest.[6] Such a duty, especially when dealing with decisions where life and the quality thereof hang in the balance, is not one to be
taken lightly. To be sure, one may choose not to fill out any type of advance
directive after going through the advance care planning process. So, too, one

may fill out one or both types of directives. It is completely up to the individual. Regardless of the type of advance directive, it does not go into effect until the patient is incompetent. Even if the patient has undergone a period of incapacity wherein his living will and/or durable power of attorney for health care guided the medical decision-making process, if the patient is later deemed competent, then decision-making authority is shifted back to the patient.

The same value underlies both the legal and moral support for advance care planning/patient autonomy. Just as autonomy drives the moral case for patient participation in medical decision-making in general[7] and advance care planning specifically, it also underlies the legal argument. Legal support for advance care planning is manifest in cases like Quinlan, Brophy, Schiavo, and most clearly in Cruzan.[8] As Ulrich maintains, "Had [Cruzan] executed a written advance directive, her case would never have gone beyond the initial court hearing and, very likely, would not have had to go to a hearing at all" (Ulrich 1999, 222). These cases stand in support of the claim that "the decisions of the courts, though not always consistent in every detail, have nonetheless emphasized the importance and role of patient self-determination in the decisional process in clinical situations" (Ulrich 1999, 39). In short, control over medical decision making ought to rest, in large part, with the patient.[9] Going further to vest decision-making authority with the patient, supporters of advance directives maintain that such authority ought to be an option for a patient even during incompetence.

The process through which advance directives were developed was not easy. Though the first model living will was put forth in 1967, with legislation supporting it introduced in the Florida State Legislature the following year; the legislation was defeated not once but twice—in 1968 and then again in 1973 (Webb 1999, 171). Not too long after, the Natural Death Act (NDA), legislation calling for the legalization of living wills, was defeated (1974) and then passed (1976) by the California state senate, making California "the first state to legalize a form of advance directive" (Webb 1999, 171). Webb does a nice job encapsulating the evolution of advance directives:

> The Quinlan decision . . . set in motion the development of a whole new body of laws that subsequently led to the U.S. Supreme Court's Cruzan decision and helped form legislation that has collectively come to be called *advance directives*. Together these laws would outline—jurisdiction by jurisdiction—how patients' decisions on their end-of-life treatment and care might be made, who should make decisions should the patient not be able to make them, and how these decisions might be implemented. (Webb 1999, 170)

Ultimately, the early 1990s brought legalization of at least some form of advance directive by all fifty states.[10]

ADVANCE DIRECTIVES: AN INTERNATIONAL VIEW

As appealing as the idea of an advance directive is, these documents are largely found in of the United States, Canada, and Europe. In a study of German doctors and judges that dealt with, among other things, attitudes on advance directives, an overwhelming majority of both physicians and judges regarded advance directives as valuable tools in determining the "presumed will" of the patient when the patient can no longer give voice to that will (van Oorschot et al. 2006). Reasons given as to why advance directives were viewed as valuable included the idea that advance directives "disburden the doctor and relatives in their decision" (therefore helping to facilitate decision making), and that they served as "communication aids" (van Oorschot et al. 2006, 624–25). While advance directives garner extensive support in Germany at present, just fifteen years ago such support was lacking at best. As van Oorschot et al. explain, as recently as 1993, the German Medical Association held that advance directives "May present simple solutions from the legal point of view; however, from the ethical and medical points of view they are no appreciable relief" (van Oorschot et al. 2006, 623). This line of thinking shifted by the late 1990s and, in 2003, advance directives were described in a German federal court case as "expression[s] of the patient's continual right to self-determination and as such being binding for doctor's and guardians" (van Oorschot et al. 2006, 623). Similarly, legal teeth were put into advance directives in Australia, where such directives have been granted "statutory status" (Parker et al. 2007).

Studies done with Finish doctors revealed a similar, positive view of advance directives. Hilden et al., in their study of over 400 Finish physicians, found that 92 percent of respondents "had a moderately or highly positive attitude toward living wills," while only 2 percent of respondents "had a moderately or highly negative attitude" (Hilden et al. 2004, 363). Even more, respondents noted important benefits that they thought were afforded by living wills. Topping the list was the promotion of patient autonomy, followed by the idea that discussing advance directives would "act as an ice breaker in discussing end of life treatment," and the belief that advance directives make decision making easier and decrease the stress so often associated with decision making at the end of life (Hilden et al. 2004, 363). Both the positive attitudes toward and the values driving such attitudes on advance directives in the countries discussed above matched those found in the United States. However, while advance directives have gained statutory residence in countries such as "Denmark, Germany, the Netherlands, New Zealand and some of the Australian and Canadian jurisdictions," in other "common law jurisdictions (including Hong Kong), there is reluctance to give advance directives greater force in law by legislation" (Chan 2004, 93). Other countries such as France, Spain, and Britain passed "living will" laws only after the turn of the century (Rosenthal 2007, 1). Thus the practice of giving legal force to advance directives, while decades old in the United States, is something relatively new to some European countries, and nonexistent in other countries.

While Browne and Sullivan, in their discussion on advance directives in Canada, claim that "there can be no serious question that making legal provisions for proxy and instructional directives is a good thing," countries all over the world are raising such questions (Browne et al. 2006, 256). Further, these questions need to be taken seriously in order to ensure that if and when the time comes that countries are ready to support advance directives through legislation, the process will be as smooth as possible. Even in countries where the discussion has progressed to include talk of advance directives gaining statutory status, the road to such status has not been easy. As one recent headline in the *International Herald Tribune* states, "Europeans are grappling with right-to-die issue; Living wills arrive, but resistance mounts" (Rosenthal 2007, 1). For example, in Italy, where advance directives are not legally recognized, physicians hold a lot of power in making medical decisions. How much or how little the patient and family are involved in the decision-making process is, in large part, up to the physician. As one Italian physician noted, "In Italy, we don't have advance directives; it is not a concept for us. . . . We think it is awkward to ask patients too far in advance whether they would want to be resuscitated. It would depend, wouldn't it, on the circumstances?" (Ripamonti 1999, 10).

While it is not imperative that the physician and patient engage in a conversation in which the patient provides the physician with details on which medical treatments he would and would not want at the end of life, it is important that the patient understands what the illness he has will "look like" in his life. That is, the patient should know when it is time to get his affairs in order, summon relatives he would want around him during his last days, decide whether or not to take a trip out of country that he has been planning with his wife; it is these things that are what will matter most in readying a patient for death.[11] The job of the physician is not necessarily to overwhelm the patient with a battery of details regarding the pathophysiological progression of the illness. Rather, it is to help the patient understand his illness and how it translates into his life narrative.

Given the wide variation in views on what "planning" for death and living at the end of life should look like, it is no wonder that advance directives have not gained residence in many places. However, this lack of acceptance of advance directives should not preclude an acceptance of the advance care planning process. For advance directives are neither a necessary nor a sufficient condition of the advance care planning process. Properly understood, advance care planning ought not focus exclusively on making decisions on particular medical treatments years in advance. Instead, it should be viewed as an opportunity for patient and provider to discuss the values that are given priority in the patient's life, how such values are understood by the patient, and how they might operate in guiding the medical treatment decisions for the patient if and when the patient becomes incompetent. Far from locking a patient into a decision, such a process can help enhance communication with his health care provider, making difficult discussions a bit easier and providing a baseline against which treatment options can compared. In short, while advance directives have not become established in several countries, the advance care planning process is something that can compliment the practice of medicine in these same countries, and enhance the communication between patient and provider. Thus, the *process* of advance care planning should be emphasized, and the skills providers need to engage in such discussions should be honed.

As another example of how advance directives are viewed, in the Netherlands while "people do sign advance directives . . . doctors are not required to comply with them" (Zylicz 1999, 12). That is, physicians have discretion as to whether or not to follow the instructions delineated in an advance directive. To truly understand the place of advance directives in the Netherlands (and anywhere else for that matter) it is crucial to understand the healthcare system and the place of a dying patient in that system more broadly.[12] In the Netherlands,

> much end-of-life care is provided by general practitioners and district nurses. They are the most important part of the health care system for these dying patients and their families. . . . This family doctor knows the patient's priorities and ways of coping. . . . Older people live in the same communities and have the same doctor for twenty years. Their physicians rely on this long-standing relationship and knowledge. (Zylicz 1999, 13)

Such in-depth knowledge of patients is a luxury. To be sure, the growing distance between patient and provider, the lack of long-term relationships in the health care context, helped drive the development of advance directives in the United States. A prime goal of advance directives is to help make sure that the patient maintains a voice in his medical treatment even after he becomes incompetent—even when being treated by health care professionals who are not familiar with him. Such directives are a way of making his voice heard, making his priorities known in a situation in which he is in the hands of strangers in what is probably an unfamiliar setting.

Despite the fact that the relationship between patient and provider is usually more established in the Netherlands as compared to the United States, there is still an important place for advance care planning. As was stated earlier, an advance directive need not evolve out of the advance care planning process, and the process is no less successful if a directive is not drafted. Rather, advance care planning needs to be viewed as a way of getting clear on a patient's preferences for care at the end of life specifically, but more generally, making manifest the values and priorities that a patient wants driving medical treatment when he is no longer competent. Making explicit patient preferences for care at the end of life is something the importance of which cannot be overemphasized. As such, assuming that these conversations will take place is at best a dangerous wager. What is at risk is losing the patient's voice at a crucial point in his own life narrative.

As Zylicz, a physician in the Netherlands, notes, the focus on the physician in caring for the patient at the end of life needs to be on the quality of life:

> You can do many things to the patient, for example, control pain, but cause loss of the ability to drive a car. In that case, the patient has no pain but cannot drive a car to visit his or her daughter. In my opinion, you cannot start palliative care soon enough and this will require talking with patients about what losses they are willing to accept and which losses they want to prevent. The patient should set the agenda. (1999, 13)

What Zylicz describes here is the very essence of advance care planning—engaging in a discussion with your patient about what is of value to him, how he defines a benefit, what burdens he is willing to bear—these issues are at the heart of the conversations that are a fundamental part of the advance care planning process. Thus, while advance directives may not have found the same legislative import that they have in the United States, it is clear that the process of advance care planning is not any less important in the Netherlands. By focusing on the documents that may or may not develop out of the advance care planning process, one is liable to overlook the great value of a good advance care planning process.[13] With that being said, advance directives have their difficulties that must be addressed prior to embarking on drafting one.

PRACTICAL DIFFICULTIES OF ADVANCE DIRECTIVES[14]: WHO IS GOING TO BEGIN THE DISCUSSION?

Advance directives are but one small part of the overall advance care planning process, yet they have garnered much of the attention. Physicians and patients alike praise their virtues. When the Patient Self-Determination Act (PSDA) was passed in 1990 (enacted in 1991), it became mandatory for all hospitals and health care providers reimbursed by Medicare and/or Medicaid to inform patients about advance directives and their rights regarding these documents. As Shewchuk explains, the pertinent standard, according to the Joint Commission on Accreditation of Healthcare Organizations, Comprehensive Accreditation Manual for Hospitals, The Official Handbook RI-11, is evaluated, for the most part, by the following "Example of Implementation":

> The hospital's policies and procedures require that a patient be told his or her right to make advance directives. The discussion is facilitated by authorized staff members who have specific training in this area or by the attending physician. The course of discussion, including any educational materials used, and its outcome are documented in the medical record. The patient or surrogate decision maker may review and modify the advance directives at any time throughout the episode of care. (Shewchuk 1998, 16)

Several factors served as driving forces behind the development and subsequent implementation of the PSDA. In general,

> The Patient Self-Determination Act provides the occasion for individuals to address many of the issues raised by their finitude as they face choices in healthcare. In order to make self-determining decisions that take the form of treatment consents, refusals, or advance directives when faced with death, disease, uncertainties, risks, etc., individuals must be aware of their values and priorities. That is, they must develop the power of reflection as it relates to their sense of self and the goals they wish to pursue in their lives. Careful attention to the Patient Self-Determination Act can help patients consider and select the time and manner of their death and the strategies to cope with the dying process. It provides a context for understanding the role of disease and injury in patients' lives. . . . [a] perspective on weighing uncertainties and risks as healthcare decisions are being considered . . . [and] help patients realize that they must face limitations in the resources available to them. (Ulrich 1999, 87)

The PSDA mandates only that patients be *informed* of their rights surrounding advance directives. Ensuring that the PSDA can help individuals realize the lofty goals above, and do so against a backdrop of cultural diversity in the clinical setting, is where the focus needs to shift in order to achieve the noble intent behind this act.

Despite the law, advance directives have yet to become entrenched in common medical practice. Why is this? What is it that is holding people back from completing advance directives? As Leahman asks, "Why are we still dying in places we would not choose, in ways we do not want, surrounded by strangers, our wishes undocumented, unknown and, therefore, often not honored?" (Leahman 2004, 249). There are several reasons why,

despite a large amount of support, the completion rate of advance directives is relatively low and, more importantly, advance care planning in
general is engaged in all too infrequently. First, health care providers, those
in the business of saving lives, may be less comfortable broaching the topic
of death as opposed to determining various ways to continue living. In addition, physicians may be concerned that discussions common to advance
care planning would increase the level of anxiety both for their patients
who are facing serious illness and those who are not. As such, the advance
care planning process is often delayed until the patient is terminally ill—if
it is initiated at all. However, this concern appears unfounded. For instance,
research on the effect discussions about CPR preference (one component
frequently touched on in advance care planning) had on the stress and
anxiety level of participants revealed "no negative effects, no increase at
all in death anxiety, anxiety, depression, or sense of control and satisfaction
with health care" (Cotton 1993, 322). In light of this type of finding, more
education needs to be focused on helping physicians become comfortable
engaging in advance care planning and training them how to do so in a way
that allows for patients to take a lead role in directing the conversations. To
be sure, not all patients will want to participate in advance care planning,
but presenting the option to do so, in a respectful and sensitive way, is a
laudable goal.

Another reason why the PSDA has not met with the great success expected
of it is because while the intention behind the act was laudable, more has to be
done in order to achieve such worthy ends. As Perkins et al. maintain, "Physicians should make advance care planning a priority in their patient care. . . .
For advance care planning to succeed, physicians must commit to it whole-
heartedly" (Perkins et al. 2002, 56). For instance, information on advance
directives given to a patient per the PSDA is often conveyed upon admission,
rather than say, by a physician during the course of a routine office visit. Even
if this information was covered in detail (which is often not the case), giving patients and families information at this chaotic time is not a good idea.
The patient is probably in a strange environment, facing new and potentially
frightening possibilities. Given such conditions, it would be more surprising
if a patient understood and appreciated the information given to him at that
time than it would be to find that such information had fallen on deaf ears. A
better time to provide patients with this information needs to be determined.
For instance, giving patients the information before admission allows them
time to go over it and include friends and loved ones. Ultimately, even if a
patient chooses not to complete an advance directive, he will be more likely
to have gained some insight into some of the foreign, opaque situations that
may arise at the end of life.

Clearly, the PSDA has not achieved its intended goal. With the current focus of medicine on trying to help as many as possible as quickly as possible, a relaxed office visit to discuss advance care planning, while seemingly a sort of pipe dream, is a promising solution. And, as reported in a follow-up study presented in 1993 at the American Geriatrics Society in Washington D.C., "there definitely are potential negative effects of not having [such discussions] because people might be resuscitated who do not want to be. . . . We showed that there isn't any harm in talking to people about it before they needed to, so the message is, talk to people" (Cotton 1993, 322). This message, though important, needs to be amended. The new message needs to be "talk to people *in a culturally sensitive manner.*"

THE PROBLEM OF UNCERTAINTY
CONCERNING THE FUTURE

Another frequent criticism of advance directives is that there is no way that a patient could take into account all of the conditions she might find herself in were she to become incompetent. Even more, determining whether such conditions would or would not be acceptable is an even more difficult task.[15] In response to these charges individuals have developed modified directives. For example, the Medical Directive,[16] developed by Linda and Ezekiel Emanuel, provides patients with parameters within which to make their medical treatment decisions (Emanuel et al. 1989). The Medical Directive is quite comprehensive, including sections on designating a health care proxy all the way to denoting preferences regarding organ donation. It also provides patients with concrete cases against which to make judgments and in light of which to form preferences regarding end-of-life care. It also has a section in which a patient can write a personal narrative. This section allows patients to provide context to his preferences and flesh out important details regarding his values (e.g., explain why he has chosen to accept or refuse particular treatments or why he has deemed a particular quality of life to be acceptable and "worth fighting for").[17] Affording patients with an opportunity to really think about their preferences and derive reasons for choosing as they do is in line with the observation Joan Teno makes in claiming that "[advance] directives with only specific instructions 'are not very helpful. . . . What is helpful is having a conversation, talking about goals and values, and concerns about dying'" (as cited in Cotton 1993, 322).[18]

In an effort to address the charges of ambiguity waged against advance directives, excellent work has been done to develop disease-specific advance directives. Voltz et al. support the utility of such directives, stating that "Advance directives should contain disease-specific information, rather than general statements that do not help in the actual clinical situation, and should be seen as part of a more general plan for end-of-life decisions in which improved communication would be more important than just the completion of a document" (Voltz et al. 1998, 154). Patients with particular diseases have a privileged perspective insofar as they have information on what the course of their disease might look like, typical ailments associated with the disease, and outcome data regarding various therapies used in treating the disease. All of this information can help to inform the advance care planning process. Further, such directives buttress the move toward more outcome- or goal-oriented advance directives. That is, as opposed to treatment-based directives that typically set out which treatments are to be administered and which are not, outcome-based directives center on demarcating the outcomes which the patient would and would not find acceptable, creating a picture of the quality of life a patient would deem to be worth pursuing. Focusing on the goals of care as opposed to specific preferences regarding specific treatments helps to avoid the criticism that advance directives ask individuals to express preferences about hypothetical health situations and treatments with which patients have little to no experience. That is, while individuals may not have any idea of what life tethered to a ventilator would "look" like, or what being dependent on a dialysis machine would mean for their daily lives, they are able to develop a picture of what a good life would look like. Even more importantly, they might be better able to sketch a picture of conditions that would not allow them to pursue their own conception of a good life. Specifically, Berry and Singer have developed the Cancer-Specific advance directive.[19] In their article, Berry and Singer lend further support to usefulness of outcome-oriented advance directives, recommending that discussions during advance care planning focus on "health states": "Health states and severity of illness have a greater influence on preferences than do treatments" (Berry and Singer 1998, 1575). In other words, what is motivating people in terms of their treatment preferences is often not concerns about the specific medical treatments rendered as much as concerns about the condition of the patient after treatment has been delivered. Thus, outcome-based advance directives seem more likely to achieve the primary purpose for which advance directives were created; to serve as vehicles through which individuals can project their values, wishes, and goals into the future and avoid being maintained in conditions that are not congruent with their conception of a good life.

A movement towards implementation of more outcome-based advance directives (both in general and for patients dealing with chronic diseases) would provide patients with a better model for expressing their wishes and greater assistance for those charged with the difficult duty of interpreting the wishes expressed in an advance directive. To be sure, gaining such knowledge of individual patients, their views on quality of life, and the things they feel are important will take time. By investing time and engaging patients in a meaningful conversation about their future health care decisions, a worthy return could be paid insofar as helping to avoid some of the burden so often experienced by those involved in making difficult health care decisions for incompetent patients.

THE PROBLEM OF COMPLETION: A FOCUS ON PROCESS

As noted earlier, while the advance care planning process might result in the drafting of an advance directive, drafting a directive is neither a necessary nor sufficient condition to procure the benefits of the process. Thus, when initiating the advance care planning process, one ought not set the drafting of a directive as a criterion for good advance care planning. In fact, many of the benefits that develop out of the advance care planning process are found in the discussions which aim toward clarifying the values pertinent to medical decision making at the end of life. Such discussions have both intrinsic and instrumental value. They are instrumentally valuable as a means to derive important information concerning values clarification and identifying the seat for decision-making authority. They are inherently valuable in that they provide individuals with the opportunity to "tell their story." There is enormous therapeutic value in being heard. Having a chance to explore and examine what it is that one holds most dear, what gives value to a life, is something the value of which cannot be overemphasized. Overall, advance care planning, when done well, is not a single, isolated event; it is a process. The edification and epiphanies that result from discussions in advance care planning are priceless resources in facilitating care at the end of life. Praise for advance care planning and recognition of the noble intent behind the PSDA are things that are well deserved—especially in Western society where autonomy reigns supreme.

What's Culture Got to Do with It?

Advance directives and advance planning are so much a part of Western culture in general that medical and legal journals both regularly "admonish" their readers that their respective patients and clients "need advance directives, including living wills" (Fagerlin and Schneider 2004, 31). However, this attitude is not universal across cultures.[20] In fact, the primacy of the main value driving advance directives, patient autonomy, is a concept that is not valued as highly in some cultures, and in others may not even make sense. While biomedicine views advance care planning as an empowering process through which an individual is able to define her own conception of a good life, and to make clear what values should guide the medical decision-making process, others may perceive it as invasive and a violation of deeply held cultural tenets. For instance, given a history of severe missteps and exploitation in medicine, it is not surprising that African Americans have not developed faith in the promise that advance directives want to make—to further patient autonomy and ensure that patient preferences will be the guiding determinant in developing a treatment plan when the patient is no longer competent. Instead, "Negative historical events lead African Americans to believe that an advance directive is equivalent to a death warrant instead of the right to freedom to ask for the health care they need and desire" (Waters 2001, 386). Studies have shown not only that culture is a predictor in determining whether an individual has an advance directive, but also whether individuals even have a desire to complete one.[21] Marshall et al. note, "only 25 percent of the African-American population, compared to 86 percent of the Euro American population, reported a desire to complete an advance directive" (Marshall et al., as cited in Swota 2008, 121). In one study with a Navajo population, not only were advance directives not desired by participants, but "86 percent of the individuals interviewed considered discussion of advance care planning for near-death medical decisions *a dangerous violation of Navajo values*" (Marshall et al. 1998, as cited in Swota 2008, 121). Given these Navajo views on speaking in a "negative way," "When the Indian Health Service adopted the requirements of the PSDA, they added the following proviso to their statutorily mandated disclosures: 'Tribal customs and traditional beliefs that relate to death and dying will be respected to the extent possible when providing information to patients on these issues'" (Zimring 2001, 23).

In addition to the conflicts that might arise concerning the values that underlie advance directives and advance care planning in general, there is a more basic problem—a disparity of knowledge about such directives. Even more, knowledge gaps between different cultural groups are not insignificant. For instance, in a survey of elderly Hispanic and white individuals, The New Mexico Elder Health Study showed that "Hispanics were less likely to correctly define a living will or durable power of attorney. Of the 70 percent of Hispanic men and women who reported that they knew what advance directives were, less than one-half had signed one compared with 60 percent of whites who had similar knowledge" (Demons and Velez 2005, 155). Thus, not only did the elderly white group know more about advance directives, but they also completed directives more frequently.[22]

Clearly, the difference in completion rates of advance directives is tied to more factors than a lack of knowledge and awareness surrounding the documents. Even under conditions in which people "speak the same language, live in the same neighborhood, attend the same community events, and share similar values . . . disagreements over moral practice can be particularly difficult to negotiate when individuals are informed by markedly distinct substantive moral norms" (Hern et al., as cited in Turner 2003, 104). In short, compounding the differences in overall awareness of advance directives are fundamental differences in values and the ways in which death and illness are approached. It is here, in a mass of different guiding norms, punctuated by different customs and practices, overlain with a thick layer of disparate languages, that the thorniest difficulties in engaging in advance care planning lie.

Understanding Autonomy

Regardless of the view one may take concerning advance directives, it is clear that the Western understanding is but one of many. The same value—autonomy—that is exalted in Western societies might not be viewed as liberating and powerful, but rather onerous and divisive, in other societies. Ekblad et al., in their study on cultural issues in hospice care in Sweden, noted that cultural clashes frequently stemmed at least in part from a difference between,

> individual and group/family oriented thinking. In an individual-oriented society, concepts like individual rights, integrity and self-determination are important. In a group-oriented society, on the other hand, the individual person is affirmed via his or her family and relatives; the individual is dependent on others in the group and also has obligations to group members. (Ekblad et al. 2000, 627)

Cultures that elevate the interconnectedness of the individual over an atomistic conception might have difficulty at a very fundamental level simply making sense of questions concerning the preferences of the individual as something separate from the group/family. Thus, the same conversations involved in advance care planning that are viewed as inclusive and comforting on a Western view, from another perspective may be construed as nonsensical or even harmful. In short, the emphasis on advance care planning in general and advance directives in particular presupposes a very specific perspective, one not shared by all and one that, if held to dogmatically, might set the stage for a rocky relationship between patients and their health care providers and institutions. If the PSDA is to function properly and attempting to engage individuals in advance care planning is to be a fruitful endeavor, those who are doing the approaching must do so in a culturally sensitive manner.

The following case illustrates how different weightings of patient autonomy and dissonant expectations of the role of the physician and patient in the medical decision-making process can generate tension and confusion between patient and provider:

Mr. Habid, an Iranian man with a complicated medical history and multiple co-morbidities went for a first appointment with a new physician, Dr. Jonas. Upon reviewing Mr. Habid's medical chart, Dr. Jonas notes the degenerative nature of a few of Mr. Habid's ailments and determines that this would be a good time to engage Mr. Habid in a discussion about advance care planning in general and advance directives in particular. After going over Mr. Habid's medical history, Dr. Jonas begins to broach the topic of advance directives. Unsure as to what such directives were, Mr. Habid asked for more information on the documents. After hearing a bit about them and skimming over the written materials Dr. Jonas had given him, Mr. Habid's demeanor changed. Both he and his wife, who had come with him to the appointment, became a bit apprehensive and developed puzzled looks on their faces. The physician noticed these change and asked the Habids if they have any questions or concerns. After a few minutes, Mr. Habid asked how long Dr. Jonas had been practicing medicine and whether he would be able to care for him given his complicated medical history. Dr. Jonas was taken aback, having viewed such questions as indicating a lack of trust. He reassured the Habids that he had exceptional training and many years of experience working with patients with complicated medical conditions. In addition, Dr. Jonas made it clear that the Habids were more than welcome to go to a different physician. For the remainder of the visit the atmosphere was strained and tense. This is in direct opposition to the calm, easy-going environment that was present at the start of the visit. After the visit Dr. Jonas was unsure what had spurred this lack of confidence and uncertainty. At the same time, Mr. Habid was not sure whether he would continue seeing Dr. Jonas.

What happened to upset the relationship that was being forged between Dr. Jonas and the Habids? Information crucial to answering this question is that Mr. Habid is originally from Iran and has been in the United States for just over three years. In some Middle Eastern cultures it is not uncommon to defer to the physician, vesting medical decision-making authority with the professional (Galanti 2003, 33). For the physician to ask what Mr. Habid would want in light of various medical scenarios was strange—shouldn't the physician know what to do and take it upon himself to make these decisions? Dr. Jonas, in looking to Mr. Habid to make such decisions as opposed to simply taking charge and making them himself, did something that troubled the Habids deeply. Since the Habids thought that medical decision making should rest solely with the expert—the physician—they construed this invitation into the decision-making process to be tantamount to the physician admitting uncertainty regarding how to treat Mr. Habid. Questioning Dr. Jonas regarding his medical training was Mr. Habid's way of trying to find reassurance that he was in good, competent medical hands. Conversely, Dr. Jonas acted in a way that he thought would maximize patient autonomy, providing Mr. Habid with an opportunity to participate in his medical treatment plan. Far from disconcerting, Dr. Jonas thought that his actions would be reassuring and reveal his deeply held belief that patients ought to be active participants in their own medical care plan. Unfortunately, given the Habid's vastly different take on the role of the patient in the medical decision-making process and the priority (or lack thereof) of patient autonomy, instead of providing a sense of empowerment to his patient, Dr. Jonas raised doubts and concerns.

This exchange may have shaken the foundation of trust between the physician and patient so deeply that a future relationship between the two may not be possible. Working toward avoiding such a consequence, Dr. Jonas could have probed more to find out why the Habids looked so perplexed and worked to provide a bit of context for his patient by explaining why such questions are asked in the context of biomedicine, and that it is standard practice to ask for the patient's participation in medical decision making. Recognizing a need to provide such reasons is an integral part of providing culturally sensitive care. Culturally sensitive providers are aware that the presuppositions and expectations of one culture are often much different than those of another culture. As such, explaining the rationale behind doing tests and asking questions will help to establish a foundation of understanding between patients and providers. This will help to ensure that differences that might arise are not due to a lack of understanding, but rather, differences in basic values and how they are prioritized.[23] Providing this extra information may have reassured Mr. Habid that soliciting his participation was not indicative of a lack of certitude when it comes to medical decision making. At the same time, Mr. Habid could have gone further to explain that in his culture, it was the role of the physician to make medical decisions. To be sure, a basic presumption of the PSDA—that individuals want and thus should have the right to have and maintain a voice in the medical decision-making process even after they become incompetent—is not shared by everyone. As Zimring explains, "there is no reason on the face of it, to think that ethical principles developed . . . from the Hippocratic tradition in medicine will be important or even present in non-western cultures" (Zimring 2001, 242).

Dr. Jonas and the Habids were working off of two disparate conceptions of autonomy. What was enhancing autonomy to Dr. Jonas—actively soliciting patient involvement in decisions regarding future medical care—was disconcerting and inappropriate to the Habids. In addition, the lofty position Dr. Jonas granted to autonomy was dramatically different than the lower priority granted to autonomy on the Habid's value hierarchy. The conflict that arose in this case may have been avoided had the physician been sensitive to the fact that there are several different ways in which people prioritize values, and that to elevate one's own ranking may result in the type of conflict Dr. Jonas ran into with the Habids. As Turner rightly points out, "For over thirty years, North American lawyers and philosophers have emphasized the principle of respect for patient autonomy and the duty to disclose, and much less attention has been directed toward how these norms of communication can be construed as disturbing, inappropriate, or morally offensive within some cultural contexts" (Turner 2003, 107).

As important as how one prioritizes autonomy is how one understands the concept. If autonomy is to continue to function and make meaningful contributions to the clinical context, it needs to take into account the diversity of the population within which it operates. Clinicians need to recognize that the Western European-American conception of the individual as "autonomous, egalitarian, rational, self-assertive, and self-aware" is but one of many (Kawaga-Singer and Kassim-Lakha 2003, 580). More specifically, it seems as though it is not necessarily the case that autonomy is a value that gets lost in translation when working across cultures. Rather, it is a value, just like beneficence and veracity, which must be construed broadly in order to function in a pluralistic setting. For example, at the start of autonomy's rise to power, it was thought that in order to act autonomously a patient needed to receive as much information as possible about his condition in a completely unbiased way (as if this is even possible), and then be left alone to make a treatment decision. To be sure, such a picture seems to be a cold, ascetic version of what autonomy might look like in practice. Even more, it does not reflect accurately the way important decisions are normally faced—within the context of relationships. A more robust conception of autonomy, one which allows for the inclusion of family and friends, and, dare I say, health care practitioners in the medical decision-making process, is one that seems to be much more useful, especially given the culturally diverse landscape one finds in the clinical setting. In other words, there is a valuable place for people other than the patient in the decision-making process. Allowing for others to take part in such a process does not take away from the autonomy of the patient, but rather, can serve to enhance it. Family members can help flesh out the values that their loved ones are trying to incorporate into the decision-making process. Health care providers can help patients and families understand the enormous amount of complex medical information so often thrust on individuals in the clinical arena. So too, health care providers should not be precluded from sharing their values that are pertinent to the decision.[24] Transparency and openness are crucial to a provider's successful divulgence of her own values and normative suggestions on how to proceed in the medical decision-making process. Understanding autonomy in relational terms, that is, "Autonomy in relation to family, culture, and the physician," is a conception that "sinks or swims depending on the development of trust and the sharing of expertise among all those involved" (Quill 2002, 232). As Quill rightly points out, the patient and family offer expertise regarding their values within the context of their culture, while the health care provider is "expert and interpreter about the culture of medicine and what it has to offer in the patient's unique circumstances" (Quill 2002, 232). With this understanding of autonomy, it is clear that rather than an isolated, individualistic decision-making process, there are a number of people involved in enhancing and facilitating a patient's opportunity to make an autonomous decision.

Overall, how one understands and prioritizes different values is tied to one's culture, one's identity. It is imperative that in order to understand patients and truly work toward patient- and family-centered medicine, those working in health care gain an understanding of cultural sensitivity and how to practice culturally sensitive health care. Gaining such an understanding and exploring various ways to effectuate different means of increasing cultural sensitivity in the fast-paced, ever-changing clinical setting will be the focus of the rest of the book. Specifically, while this project is merely a start to a process that will require continuous work and attention, it is a useful first step in helping to offer patients the opportunity to engage in a culturally sensitive health care experience, particularly a culturally sensitive advance care planning process.

NOTES

1. Again, I want to focus on this model as it operates in the clinical setting.

2. Other cases pivotal in molding the concept of informed consent and its place in U.S. law include *Salgo v. Leland Stanford Jr. University* (1957), *Natanson v. Kline* (1960), *Canterbury v. Spence* (1972), and *Cobbs v. Grant* (1972).

3. There is not unanimity regarding the view that informed consent is a useful and important component of the provider-patient relationship. As Kettle describes, "Although ethical necessity is obvious to proponents of informed consent, practicing clinicians are at most halfhearted about it. . . . Even those clinicians who are committed to informed consent are unclear about how to use it at the bedside" (Kettle 2003, 43). This lack of acceptance by health care providers may stem, in part, from the fact that informed consent requirements were born out of the law and thrust onto medicine, rather than evolving out of a need noted within medicine and addressed by health care professionals (see Katz in Steinbock et al. 2003). The value of informed consent in the clinical provider-patient relationship is a question that exceeds the scope of this book. For more on this debate see O'Neill 2001.

4. I will use the term "informed consent" when speaking of a valid consent, though it is equally as important to be informed when making a valid refusal.

5. I will use the term "surrogate" hereafter.

6. As Ulrich explains:

While "substituted judgment" attempts to replicate the wishes of the incompetent, the "best interest" standard makes no substantial reference to the wishes of the incompetent. . . . Instead, the best-interest standard assumes the position of a "reasonable" observer who weighs all of the factors in the patient's situation and makes a decision (albeit based on an evaluation and balancing of factors involved) that is deemed to promote the best interest of the patient. (Ulrich 1999, 43)

7. For instance, autonomy drives informed consent requirements that are so integral to daily clinical practices.

8. These are just a few of the many decisions in which courts have been clear in their support of allowing the values of individuals (planning for health care in case of a future which may encompass their incompetence), either expressed by the individual or by a surrogate, to guide decision making in the medical treatment plan.

9. The accolades for ACP also include being heralded as a process that can help facilitate (as much as is possible) navigation of the often complex terrain involved in end-of-life decision making. Murray and Jennings maintain, "the system of end of life care in general works best for those who plan ahead for their terminal illness, and it does not always work well even for them" (Murray and Jennings 2005, S53).

10. As Webb explains:

Different state laws varied not only on whether they were living will or health-care proxy laws, but *when* they applied (for example, some states allow them to cover only terminally ill; some include those in persistent vegetative states; some exclude pregnant women), *who* could decide for a patient not able to decide for himself or herself, and *how* that decision might be made. (1999, 173)

For the specific parameters of legislation in different jurisdictions, one may refer to the Wall Street Journal piece, "Advance Directives by State," March 22, 2005. Found at online.wsj.com/public/article/SB111144394604885495-4MQpLbfZZSZWMXQ4BdPaL0_1d0k_20050421.html?mod=tff_main_tff_top. Accessed April 22, 2008.

11. If the patient chooses to have this information given to someone else, that is also acceptable. The important point is that the patient makes that decision. I will say more about this in chapter 4.

12. An in-depth understanding of the healthcare systems in each of the countries mentioned in this book is far beyond the scope of this project. Simply being aware of the intricate connection between the take on advance directives and the health care system at issue is a necessary starting point to developing a sense of why or why not such directives are accepted.

13. To be sure, in many jurisdictions in the United States, an advance directive need not be written.

14. I will focus on some of the "practical" difficulties noted with advance directives (specifically living wills), as opposed to the deeper "philosophical" difficulties of

advance directives. Briefly though, one of the main philosophical difficulties regarding advance directives is how to view the incompetent patient. Ought she to be viewed as the incompetent individual she is at present, often with highly abridged interests? Or, ought she to be viewed as the competent individual she once was? The answer to this question will determine a number of important things, most fundamentally, how much weight (if any) should be given to the advance directive in the decision-making process.

15. Lynn 1991 and Fagerlin and Schneider 2004 are representative examples from a vast literature that touch on this point.

16. Though the Medical Directive (Emanuel and Emanuel 1989) is the "preferred approach" of the American Medical Association Council on Ethical and Judicial Affairs, Culver notes that there are other forms available that are superior in certain respects to the Medical Directive. Some examples include the Five Wishes (agingwithdignity.org/5wishes.html) from Aging with Dignity, Respecting Choices from Gundersen Lutheran Medical Foundation, and Caring Conversations from the Center for Practical Bioethics (State Initiatives in End-of-Life Care, issue 23, March 2005, p. 5, www.rwjf.org/files/publications/other/State_Initiatives_EOL23.pdf).

17. To be sure, there are arguments from organizations pushing for facilitating the ability of individuals to request life-sustaining treatment to be initiated and continued when and if they become incompetent. Such organizations maintain that advance directives are a means by which individuals can make such wishes known. This type of argument is made by the Robert Powell Center for Medical Ethics of the National Right to Life Committee in their report entitled "Will Your Advance Directive Be Followed?" (April 15, 2005, www.nrlc.org).

18. Another development that has served to help clarify patients' wishes regarding medical treatments and make them known to health care providers across various settings is the POLST (Physician Orders for Life-Sustaining Treatment). For more information on the "POLST Paradigm" see www.POLST.org.

19. See Berry and Singer 1998, and Singer 1997.

20. To be sure, this attitude is not universal within any one culture.

21. As one study noted, "ethnicity was the second most significant predictor of possession of an advance directive after education" (Berger as cited in Swota 2008, 121). In the context of this project, one may understand ethnicity and culture as similar constructs. See chapter 2 for a more extensive discussion of the concept of culture. See below for how I will understand ethnicity. An extended comparison between the two terms is beyond the scope of this project.

Ethnicity: Ethnicity is a social and political construct used by individuals and communities to define themselves and others. Specifically, ethnicity refers to a person's cultural background, including his or her language, origin, faith, and heritage. Ethnicity comprises the ideas, beliefs, values, and behaviour that are transmitted from one generation to the next. Ethnicity tends to be perceived in terms of common culture, history, language, or nationality. Ethnicity and ethnic identity are interchangeable terms. (www.students.ubc.ca/access/race.cfm?page=glossary, accessed September 19, 2008)

22. Much more will be said about reasons why, even when Hispanics (and other groups) know about advance directives and advance care planning in general, they are

less likely than whites to engage in the process and/or complete an advance directive.

23. To be sure, providing such a foundation is part of being a good health care provider in general.

24. For a nice model of how providers can share their values with patients, see Brody and Quill's "enhanced-autonomy" model (Brody and Quill 1996).

Chapter Two

A Plurality of Cultures

The field of bioethics faces the same problems of the need for respect for diversity as those faced in biomedicine and society in general. It must allow for a broader, more inclusive view of human needs and emotions while maintaining a sense of unity in ethical guidelines and recognition of the human condition.

—Loustaunau and Sobo (1997, 139)

As one of the nurses coming on duty approached her patient's room she could hear the wails of the new mother, a young Cambodian woman. Accompanying her sobs were the angry voices of family members at the bedside. Multiple staff members were in the room and outside the door trying to calm the family down. The nurse thought that something had happened to the couple's newborn daughter, that an unexpected ailment had befallen her and that it must have been serious to have caused the family to become so upset. After asking several staff members who had been at the patient's room since the commotion had begun, the nurse realized that the baby was "fine," not even so much as an elevated white blood cell count. What had happened was that the small string bracelet that was tied around the baby's wrist had been cut off and thrown away. The nurses thought that it might harbor germs that could wreak havoc on the child given her immature immune system. Far from a potential source of harm to her child, the Cambodian mother placed the strings known as *baci* around the child's wrist in order to "tie in the soul" to make sure that it did not "get lost" (Galanti 2004, 60). *Baci* are never supposed to be cut off, but rather "wear off in time" (Galanti 2004, 60). Cutting the strings off was an act of beneficence from the nurse's perspective, a way of decreasing the possibility of infection. From the new mother's perspective, cutting off the

33

strings represented an assault on the safety of her new baby's soul. Seemingly simple, insignificant acts can often serve to destroy the relationship between patients, families, and health care providers. To underestimate the importance of avoiding such misunderstandings is foolish at best.

Raising awareness of the fact that not all people subscribe to the tenets of the biomedical model is a necessary first step in developing a good health care provider-patient relationship. Differences in the beliefs and practices surrounding health and illness run deep and are often so imbedded in one's culture that an individual is often unaware of them. Culture is not something that "resides in the conscious mind," nor is it something of which one person has more or less than another.[1] It often operates subterraneously and has a profound impact on an individual's life. The scope of culture's influence is broad to say the least, shaping such things as one's view of religion, diet and exercise, child-rearing, familial structure, decision-making procedures, health and illness, and hierarchy of values in general. Overall, culture colors and shapes the "lens through which an individual views the world"—defining notions of common sense and inhabiting every corner of one's world view.[2]

The power and influence of culture has been described as disruptive, a sort of "distorting lens" that got in the way of seeing clearly from "the moral point of view" and the removal of which was the "task of moral philosophy" (Turner 2003, 100). It has become apparent that this lens cannot be removed—that culture is not something that can or should be factored out when considering an individual. It is an integral part of what makes a person who she is. To even attempt to "wipe away" the "distorting lens of culture" would be an effort made in vain. What is more, if it were even possible, removing the influence of culture would not clarify one's view of the world, but rather, provide an incomplete picture of how an individual sees the world. Instead of immediately trying to divorce individuals from the influence of culture, it behooves us to aim toward understanding and working within a clinical setting where very different approaches to viewing the world come together. To be sure, some cases will arise in which certain cultural practices cannot and should not be accommodated (e.g., practices that violate human rights). However, an attitude of mutual respect, in which health care providers and patients work together to develop mutually agreeable treatment options, needs to be fostered. Specifically, I want to focus on the issue of how to engage in medical decision making, particularly advance care planning, against a backdrop of cultural diversity.

It is helpful to first set out what I will take culture to mean and address some of the salient issues that arise at the intersection of culture and advance care planning. Culture is a concept that has been defined several different ways.[3] For the purposes of this text, I will use the definition put forth by

Krakauer et al., in which culture refers to "a constellation of shared meanings, values, rituals, and modes of interacting with others that determines
how people view and make sense of the world" (as cited in Werth et al. 2002,
184).[4] Other definitions of culture that help to flesh out the various nuances of
this complex concept within the health care context include the following:

> The thoughts, communications, actions, customs, beliefs, values, and institu-
> tions of racial, ethnic, religious, or social groups. Culture defines how health
> care information is received, how rights and protections are exercised, what is
> considered to be a health problem, how symptoms and concerns about the prob-
> lem are expressed, who should provide treatment for the problem, and what type
> of treatment should be given. (Bronheim and Sockalingam 2003, 4)

Taken together, these definitions provide a good indication of how complex
and robust the concept of culture truly is.

The influence of culture on how one understands health and illness, what
these things "look like" to an individual, cannot be overemphasized—it is absolutely fundamental to successful interactions in the clinical setting.[5] Briefly,
an awareness of the fact that "health" can mean more than just "freedom from
physical disease or pain" and illness more than "an unhealthy condition of
body or mind" is essential in providing culturally sensitive care (Merriam-
Webster online dictionary, entry for "health" accessed April 10, 2008, entry
for "illness" accessed April 10, 2008, www.merriam-webster.com/dictionary/
health). As Spector explains,

> health can be regarded not only as the absence of disease but also as a reward
> for "good behavior." . . . A state of health is regarded by many people as the
> reward one receives for "good" behavior, and illness as a punishment for "bad"
> behavior. . . . Health can also be viewed as the freedom from and the absence
> of evil. In this context, health is analogous to day, which equals good light. . . .
> Illness is analogous to night, evil, and dark. (Spector 2004, 49)

As such, a provider must enter into a relationship with a patient with an
open mind not only with regard to potential treatment options, for instance,
but also with regard to drastically different views on what it is to be "ill" or
"healthy." For instance, if one is taking medications for which one of the side
effects is a compromised immune system, it might seem superfluous to discuss in any great detail why it is best to minimize exposure to germs and go
over good hand washing practices. However, this belief rests on the presupposition that an individual buys into germ theory (Loustauna and Sobo 1997,
115), as opposed to, for instance, the idea that illness is a sort of "punishment"
for some unrighteous past act. Anne Fadiman, in her exemplary book *The*

Spirit Catches You and You Fall Down, provides a wonderful illustration of this point with the following case of a Hmong family:

> A child in San Diego was born with a harelip. Her doctors asked the parents' permission to repair it surgically. They cited the ease of the operation, the social ostracism to which the child would be otherwise condemned. Instead, the parents fled the hospital with their baby. Several years earlier, while the family was escaping from Laos to Thailand, the father killed a bird with a stone, but he had not done so cleanly and the bird had suffered. The spirit of the bird had caused the harelip. To refuse to accept punishment would be a grave insult. (Fadiman 1998, 262)

Not only does this case highlight the disparate beliefs people may have regarding the cause or etiology of a medical condition or illness, but it also points to the varying ideas on what constitutes an "illness" and what may be considered "treatments." More broadly, it indicates what proper "care" of an individual would look like. On the biomedical model, proper care for a harelip is surgery to correct it. For the Hmong family mentioned above, care as defined in the biomedical model translated into disrespect and an unwillingness to accept an owed punishment. Even more, to challenge the divine intervention that caused the harelip would set the child up for a fate much worse than the one described by the physicians if corrective surgery was refused. To be sure, the very notion that individuals have control over their own health (and illness) is, at the least, not a universal assumption. For many, the locus of control over health and illness rests outside of human control. Instead, it is a matter of luck or fate.[6]

Differences also surface with regard to how individuals manifest their emotions. For example, how does one react to pain or to information (good and bad) concerning her own health or the health of a loved one? Does one cower at the thought of a paper cut? Remain Stoic while having a dislocated shoulder put back into place? Cry openly in front of strangers? Not shed a tear even in the face of the death of a beloved family member? Maintain a placid demeanor when told that one's cancer is in remission? Or explode with cries of joy at the mere mention of an upcoming birth? Too often people are judged to be demonstrating "appropriate" responses to various situations—as if there is some standard measure by which they could be judged. Manifestations of happiness and sorrow, appreciation and disinterest might look very different depending upon the lens, so shaped by cultural influences, through which the situation is viewed.

Take for instance a case in which, while rounding, a health care worker overhears a group of nurses discussing the family of a patient that had been in the ICU for several days. The patient, an elderly Japanese man, was gravely ill and his prognosis was dire at best. Upon hearing the bad news about the poor prognosis, the patient's family, several of whom were at the hospital every day, nodded in recognition and moments later, picked up their previous conversation where they had left off. The nurses took this response to be lacking in "proper" emotion, evidence of an uncaring family, and generally unacceptable. How could such bad news not be met with cries of disbelief, perhaps a fainting family member, at least a single tear? In fact, the family was quite dedicated and caring. They were constantly at the patient's bedside and appreciative of the care their loved one was receiving. However, they were not very expressive, even in light of the devastating news. This lack of outward expression of grief was not indicative of apathy, or insensitivity. It was simply the way that bad news was taken in their culture. In short, it does not follow that because a family is quite demonstrative in their expression of grief that they care a great deal for their loved one who is sick. Nor does it follow that a family that is more reserved in the face of bad news cares very little about their ailing loved one. Grief is expressed (or not) in a plethora of ways. Searching for some standard measure by which to judge whether a family has expressed it (or any other emotion for that matter) in an "appropriate" manner would be an exercise in futility. Rather, recognizing such differences and suspending judgment in the absence of greater understanding is a practice that will prove more fruitful.[7]

Judgments such as the one mentioned above often arise from a stance in which, while making judgments about others, one uses "one's own standards, values, and beliefs. . . . The standards against which others are measured are understood to be superior, true, or morally correct, while those being evaluated and not 'measuring up' are inferior or wrong" (Loustauna and Sobo 1997, 14). In contrast, "cultural sensitivity can be understood as being aware of one's own culture and the biases encompassed therein, being willing to understand and be open to the beliefs and practices of different cultures, and being willing to place an emphasis on communicating in a manner amenable to everyone involved" (Swota 2008, 109). To be sure, the judgment that one's own standards are superior in a particular case may be correct. However, to simply assume such superiority based solely on the fact that they are one's own is a problem. Such a stance allows one to fall back on something familiar. Making judgments based on what one has intimate knowledge of is comfortable, and likely, reflexive. It is not surprising that such a practice has invaded the medical arena, given the diverse backdrop against which medical care and treatment decisions are being made. Reactions to this stance vary. Extremes are represented by those who held fast to the core of this practice, that one's own "way" is right and others are wrong insofar as they differ, and those that gravitated to the opposite extreme of cultural relativism. As Macklin explains, "What is the obligation of physicians in the United States when they encounter patients in such situations? At one extreme is the reply that in the United States, physicians are obligated to follow the ethical and cultural practices accepted here and have no obligation to comply with patients' requests that embody entirely different cultural values. At the other extreme is the view that cultural sensitivity requires physicians to adhere to the traditional beliefs and practices of patients who have emigrated from other cultures" (Macklin 1998, 12).[8] Macklin concludes, "We ought to be able to respect cultural diversity without having to accept every single feature embedded in traditional beliefs and rituals" (Macklin 1998, 19).

Cultural relativism (CR) is a view developed by nineteenth-century anthropologists. Prima facie, CR seems to be a very accepting and tolerant view.[9] According to CR, right and wrong are a matter of culture. Different cultures hold different ethical beliefs, and when they conflict there is no "right" answer, just different views. Overall, cultural relativists begin with the descriptive claim that different cultures have different values and beliefs. From there, the cultural relativist draws the conclusion that ethics is relative to culture (Rachels and Rachels 2006, 18–21). Thus, when making a normative judgment about a practice, one must refer to the standards set by the culture within which the practice is being performed. According to the cultural relativist, there are no objective standards of right and wrong; rightness and wrongness are whatever one's culture says is right or wrong. In other words, if a practice is deemed to be right or acceptable in a particular culture, it is right regardless of how those from other cultures judge it. The implication is that there are never any "mistakes" in the ethical practices of a culture. Swallowing such an implication would be difficult at best. As such, "The challenge for clinical practice is to allow ethical pluralism — a true engagement with and respect for diverse perspectives — without falling into the trap of absolute ethical relativism" (Koenig and Gates-Williams 1995, 248).

Female genital mutilation (FGM)[10] is an example often given to highlight the consequences of an unthinking relativism. Though practiced in several countries, FGM is most common in many African and Arab nations. FGM is illegal in the United States and elsewhere. There are different types of FGM; the most common of these include a process in which the "hood of the clitoris, the clitoris itself, or the clitoris as well as both the inner and outer labia, are removed" (Loustaunau and Sobo 1997, 15).[11] After the procedure, during which the clitoris and both the inner and outer labia are removed, "the two sides of the wound [are] stitched together, leaving a small pinhole opening for the drop by drop passage of urine and menstrual blood" (Loustaunau and Sobo 1997, 15). FGM is not a benign procedure, but rather one that carries with it high risk for both immediate and long term side effects.[12] It is precisely when cultural practices encroach on territory marked by torture, grave physical and mental harm, and human rights violations, that such practices cannot, indeed must not, be accepted.[13]

Though on the face of it cultural relativism seems to be a kinder, gentler approach to viewing the world—a sort of "to each his own" mentality—upon further examination (as illustrated in the case of FGM) it is a view with dire consequences. In holding fast to cultural relativism, one is precluded from criticizing the practices of other cultures— regardless of how brutal or dehumanizing. The most that a cultural relativist can say when faced with a practice "X" in another culture that is not accepted in her own is, "In my culture 'X' is wrong, but it is 'right' in this other culture." Now, replace "X" with "violence toward homosexuals," "cruelty toward children," and "hatred of and random acts of violence against [fill in with a religious group] should be furthered." "Tolerance" of these other views seems to be morally repugnant at best. As Rachels and Rachels rightly explain, "there is nothing in the nature of tolerance that requires you to say that all beliefs . . . all social practices are equally admirable. On the contrary, if you did not think that some were better than others, there would be nothing for you to tolerate" (Rachels and Rachels 2006, 29). Acknowledging that one is wrong in one's own beliefs or values, or that another culture might have a better (or worse) approach, is a privilege that is afforded only if one rejects cultural relativism. Turner does well in summarizing this need to strike a balance between two extremes (i.e., ethical absolutism and cultural relativism), especially within the clinical setting:

> The dual dangers in addressing the moral obligations of health care providers in multicultural, pluralistic settings are those of falling into a facile acceptance of all cultural and religious norms, even when some practices cause great harm and violate basic human rights, and insisting upon a narrow understanding of acceptable moral reasoning, when there is good reason to think that a plurality of human religious and cultural practices should be accommodated. (Turner 2002, 298–99)

One way such balance might be struck is to adopt a pluralistic stance that acknowledges the idea that there is not only one "right" way of living, accommodating different cultural practices and beliefs. At the same time that pluralism recognizes the importance of trying to accommodate the views and practices of others, it also allows for criticism of one's own views and practices, and those of others. The following case serves as a nice illustration of how to accommodate different cultural practices:

> Mrs. Bahnar, a thirty-nine-year old Somali woman was admitted to the hospital with complaints of nausea, dizziness, blurred vision, and general malaise. She had been in the hospital for two days undergoing a range of diagnostic tests,

when her family began to burn incense at her bedside. Right away the nurses told her family that burning incense (or anything else for that matter) was not permissible in the hospital. The Bahnar family became extremely agitated, yelling at the nurses. Other patients and families began to complain and the nurses had to call security. Eventually, the Bahnars calmed down, but their actions and the resulting disorder stayed with the nurses. After this incident, several nurses asked not to be assigned to care for Mrs. Bahnar.

In an effort to understand what had happened, rectify the situation, and stave off further conflicts, the health care team requested that the bioethicist at the hospital come in and meet with Mrs. Bahnar and her family. The Bahnars explained to the bioethicist that burning incense is an integral part of a customary "healing ritual." Briefly,

> Somalis have a concept of spirits residing within each individual. When the spirits become angry, illnesses such as fever, headache, dizziness, and weakness can result. The illness is cured by a healing ceremony designed to appease the spirits. These ceremonies involve reading the Koran, eating special foods, and burning incense. (ethnomed.org/ethnomed/cultures/somali/somali_cp.html, accessed June 20, 2007)

The bioethicist relayed this information to the health care team and suggested that the team sit down with the Bahnar family to try and understand their request, to explain how burning incense was against the fire codes of the hospital, and to try and work out a mutually agreeable plan. Ultimately, Mrs. Bahnar was able to be wheeled out to an outdoor patio right near her room. Here, the Bahnars were allowed to burn the incense without being in violation of the fire codes. For the Bahnars, engaging in an important cultural practice put them in violation of the law. Entering into a dialogue with hospital staff to explain why they were burning the incense, and being given an explanation as to why the health care providers put a stop to it, allowed both sides to gain insight into where the other was coming from. Open communication and a sense of inquiry were invaluable tools in resolving what could have been an even more intense conflict. Even more, it allowed the Bahnars to perform important components of a traditional healing ritual—something that they saw as their familial duty to carry out. By adopting a pluralistic stance, the parties involved in this situation were able to discharge their duties and avoid violating the law—something that would not have been possible if an open and accommodating stance had not been taken by the health care team.

At a deeper level, one should not assume that differences in behavior denote differences in underlying principles. Prima facie, what might seem to be differences (sometimes even great differences), may be different practices which are driven by the same underlying values. As Jennings explains:

cultural traditions give individuals a language within which to comprehend and communicate their experience, a lens through which to perceive themselves and the world, and a repertoire of meanings and symbols with which to organize their experiences and make them cohere into some kind of whole. These traditions vary greatly on the surface, so to speak, but perhaps at a deeper level they tend to converge on some similar themes. . . . The subjects of death, dying, pain, suffering, care, dignity, and peace at the end of life may in fact lead one to that terrain where our diverse humanness recedes and our common humanity comes to the fore. (Jennings 1999, 12 of 16)

Such differences in behavior might stem not from disparate values to which individuals from different cultures subscribe, but rather, from divergent interpretations of the same values. In addition, such differences are also influenced by disparities in how individuals from different cultures weigh and prioritize values. For instance, autonomy might be given primacy in one culture and fall far behind several other values (e.g., beneficence, nonmaleficence) in another culture. Whether differences in behavior and preference are driven by adherence to vastly different values, variant interpretations of the same values, dissimilar weighting of the same values, or some other combination altogether, I want to focus on ways to increase the level of understanding of such differences and look at ways to accommodate such differences in the clinical setting; a setting that is directed, in part, by mandates that often fail to recognize the pluralistic population that they cover.

NOTES

1. Thanks to Kerry Bowman for making this point.
2. Thanks to Kerry Bowman for making this point.
3. One's "cultural makeup" consists of several components, including, but not limited to, "race, language, dialect, geographic pattern, migratory pattern, religion, employment pattern, history, art, literature, folklore, proverbs, music, food, customs, symbols, family structure, relationships, and sexual dominance" (Orr 1996, 2004).
4. Other definitions of culture include that of Perkins et al., in which culture is defined as "the values, beliefs, and behaviors that a people hold in common, transmit across generations, and use to interpret their experiences" (Perkins et al. 2002, 48). In addition, culture has been defined as "all the shared, learned knowledge that people in a society hold," where society is defined as a group of people "who share a specific geographical area within which they interact together, guided by their culture." (Loustauna and Sobo 1997, 10).
5. Kawaga-Singer and Kassim-Lakha have described culture as having two functions, the integrative and the prescriptive:

The integrative function provides individuals with the beliefs and values that provide meaning in life and a sense of identity, and the prescriptive are the rules for behavior that support an individual's sense of self-worth, and maintain group function and welfare. (2003, 578–79)

6. Thanks to Kerry Bowman for clarifying this point.

7. In an effort to understand grief and grieving, several theories have been developed. Most prominent among such theories are those known as "stage theories." These theories (most notably that of Kübler Ross) identify and describe the stages through which people pass in the grieving process. As Mulhall points out, these theories have been "criticized for being simplistic and possibly leading nurses to believe that any deviation from the path is abnormal." In addition, Mulhall contends that such theories "have been developed into a highly biomedical perspective, which contends that there are normal and abnormal grief reactions" (Mulhall 1996, 38).

8. The first "extreme" can be viewed as a sort of ethical absolutism in which "there are 'universally true' ethical principles that apply to everyone, everywhere, at all times" (Frederick 1999, 66). The opposite extreme is ethical/cultural relativism. Ethical pluralism provides a nice middle ground between the extremes of ethical absolutism and ethical relativism. For a nice overview of ethical pluralism see Timmons 2002.

9. I will be giving only a brief description of cultural relativism. There is a vast body of literature on this topic. See especially Macklin 1999.

10. Female genital mutilation is sometimes referred to as "female circumcision."

11. For a good overview of some of the different types of FGM, see Editors, "What's Culture Got to Do with it? Excising the Harmful Tradition of Female Circumcision." *Harvard Law Review*, 106 (June 1993): 1944–61.

12. "Immediate effects can include intense pain, shock, hemorrhage, retention of urine and menstrual discharge, fever, tetanus, and genital infection. The girl or woman may die if a major blood vessel is cut and she cannot reach a medical facility equipped to deal with such emergencies. . . . Post-operative ailments that can materialize intermittently during later years . . . include reproductive tract infections that sometimes are severe enough to cause infertility, urinary tract infections, cysts, and the formation of obstructive genital scar tissue" ("What's Culture Got to Do with it?" *Harvard Law Review*, 1993).

13. To be sure, in order to accept that practices that violate human rights ought not be accepted, one must first agree that there are human rights (i.e., rights individuals have simply in virtue of being human). An argument for human rights exceeds the scope of this book. For a nice overview of human rights and the issues surrounding them, see The Internet Encyclopedia of Philosophy, entry "Human Rights" at www. iep.utm.edu/h/hum-rts.htm#SH5a.

Chapter Three

Communicating Across Cultures

No one individual can anticipate all the problems that might arise in an attempt to understand chronic illness and disability in a multicultural society, but we can all have enough sensitivity to realize that there might be significant differences, and enough respect for others to ask questions and listen carefully to the replies.

—Groce and Zola

Being invited in to listen to patients tell their stories and share some of their most personal information is a privilege. When entering into a relationship with a patient, health care practitioners must remember this and focus on maintaining an open mind and strive to foster a foundation of trust with the patient. For instance, "Among many West Indian and Central American blacks, communication about an upcoming death or communication with the dead may often be revealed through dreams. Attempts at spiritual healing may be concealed from providers to avoid the stigma attached to such practices, which may be labeled as devil worshipping or mumbo-jumbo by mainstream European-American culture" (Welch 2001, 41). Welch maintains that "When such medical or health-related information is revealed, providers should place it in its proper cultural context. Insofar as possible the physician should work with the patient to accommodate personal beliefs into any treatment plan" (Welch 2001, 41). Being open to other views and never dismissing any view out of hand as silly or ignorant will afford practitioners the best chance at truly understanding the views and conditions of their patients. Even more, it will facilitate open communication and increase the chances of being invited in to be informed about a patient's preferences and values. This invitation is instrumental in successful advance care planning.

Interactions in a diverse clinical setting will benefit from health care providers becoming culturally sensitive. Becoming culturally sensitive entails gaining an awareness of one's own culture and how it shapes one's perspective, values, and biases. Understanding that there are vast differences in how people approach and deal with illness in general is imperative. However, while it is good to know about some of the ways people in other cultures might behave in the face of a poor prognosis, for example, the value of such knowledge is founded in large part on the fact that it serves to make health care providers aware of the diversity of reactions they might face in their encounters with patients. For example, it helps to drive home the idea that there is no "normal" or "standard" reactions to hearing bad news. To be sure, there are no "standard" reactions in patient encounters. In aiming toward becoming culturally sensitive, openness to diversity and a desire to understand various perspectives are crucial traits. Clinical interactions will be successful insofar as those involved in the relationship are listened to, their views respected as much as possible, and a treatment plan is created through a process in which all parties have participated and on which consensus has been obtained.

The following case provides a nice example of how health care providers, by entering into patient encounters with an open mind and a willingness to negotiate, can make patients and families feel comfortable enough to share what can prove to be valuable information, crucial to providing proper treatment. If a certain level of comfort is not established, patients and families may not provide full information to providers, compromising the health and well-being of the patient and making the job of the provider very difficult. The case comes from Perinatal Nurse Case Manager Margie Dogotch, at The Perinatal Program: A Community Health Worker Model of La Clinica del Cariño Family Health Center, Inc. Dogotch explains how providers, in trying to communicate effectively with patients, "need to understand how to talk about sensitive issues such as sexuality, drug use, and personal violence, among others. Just as importantly, the provider must learn how not to react negatively when client responses differ from one's own belief system" (Cultural Competence Works 2001). Dogotch provides the following example:

> in Hispanic culture . . . there's a strong belief about a fallen fontanel, the soft spot, when a baby's soft spot is sunken, or low around the hole in the skull, that's a bad thing, so they will hold the baby upside down by the feet and shake it a little so the hole fills back up. Medically, the Western belief is that it is sunken from dehydration. Mind you, it's not a strong shake, you just turn the baby upside down, then turn it back up again. So we don't blow that tradition off, we say, "what have you done so far, ok, you held the baby upside down, good, you need to do that, but you also need to give the baby lots of water, or breast

milk, or formula. So every time you see this, do the holding upside down, but also make sure the baby gets lots of liquids." That's the value of the information from the community being integrated into medical care. We honor and respect their beliefs and traditions, and the children are also being attended to medically. (Cultural Competence Works 2001)

As the case above points out, health care providers need to be aware of the differences that exist in dealing with illness and approaching death, and recognize that attempting to incorporate these differences into treatment plans for patients is something that is foundational to practicing medicine in a culturally sensitive manner. In fact, it is a core component of practicing good medicine in general. Prima facie it may seem quite facile to develop an awareness of the ways of others, but given that "the ways in which culture, ethnicity, race, and a host of other factors *powerfully but almost invisibly shape*[1] the interactions of patients and caregivers," such awareness might not be so easily developed (Jennings 1999, 14 of 16).

COMMUNICATION: THE TOWER OF BABBLE

One of the necessary conditions of being culturally sensitive, and most helpful in developing care plans that respect the various perspectives involved, is recognizing the importance of good patient-provider communication. To be sure, good communication is important in any patient-provider relationship, but its importance is underscored even more when engaging in the sensitive and intimate conversations that are entailed in advance care planning. One study based on data from the Medical Expenditure Panel Survey showed that "Hispanics were significantly less likely than whites to believe that their primary physician listened to them, and Asians were least satisfied with their interactions with health care staff" (Kawaga-Singer and Kassim-Lakha 2003, 584). If individuals are not being listened to, feel as though they are not being listened to, or are generally dissatisfied with their interactions with health care staff, providers will have an uphill battle in getting patients to engage in the deeply personal process of advance care planning. For a patient to feel comfortable engaging in such a personal dialogue with his health care professional, there must be a sense of trust—trust that will enable the patient to open up to his provider. It is hard to imagine that an individual would be willing to discuss his deepest values and the context within which he understands them with a provider he does not trust, or at least feels comfortable enough with to start a relationship.

Given the importance of establishing and maintaining good communication, I want to spend some time delving into ways to cultivate clear and open lines of communication. I will examine reasons why communication may become murky, leaving the provider-patient relationship open to conflict and misunderstanding. Muddled by numerous factors, a common culprit of marred communication is a language difference between patient and provider. Such differences have become quite common as an ever-increasingly diverse patient population interacts with a diverse provider population. Specifically, "More than 31 million Americans are unable to speak the same language as their health care provider" (Flores 2000, 16). To be sure, even when a patient and a provider come from the same cultural background, there is no guarantee that the patient will understand everything that is told to him. This is especially true in the fast-paced clinical setting, rife with acronyms and complex medical terminology—a language that may be inaccessible to many patients. Couple the complex language of the health care provider with the often anxious state of a sick patient, and there is even more reason to think that communication between patient and provider might not go smoothly. How can patients be expected to remain calm in the face of dire diagnoses and prognoses "communicated" to them sandwiched between requests for ABGs, potassium levels, and a variety of radiological tests? Take for example the following case in which a patient's attempt at levity was met with a literal translation—causing confusion and concern rather than lightheartedness and calm for the patient.

A nervous patient jokingly asked his surgeon if he was going to "kick the bucket." The Korean physician, wanting to reassure the patient that his upcoming surgery would be successful, responded affably, "Oh, yes, you are definitely going to kick the bucket!" (Galanti 2004, 20)

This case is an example of what Hallenbeck et al. refer to as a "cultural faux pas," in which "there is a simple misunderstanding as to the meaning of a particular action or behavior between members of different groups" (Hallenbeck et al. 1996, 395). In this case, the health care provider and patient spoke the same language, but misunderstandings created tension and discomfort. And, though the anxiety created by the provider's misinterpretation of the patient's attempt at humor can be cleared up as quickly as it was created, such added unrest is an unwelcome addition at any time, but especially right before going into surgery. Remedying the problem would entail an explanation from both the patient and the provider as to what they meant by their comments—namely, humor on the part of the patient and comfort on the part of the provider. It is important to remember though, that when engaging in something as crucial as advance care planning, the cost of confusion, especially if it is not cleared up right away, may be a lost opportunity for an individual to retain a voice in her medical treatment. So too, it might also mean a confused and ambiguous directive is produced that muddies the decision-making waters rather than adding clarity. Potentially, it could deter a patient from even attempting to engage in advance care planning at all. Ultimately, if nothing else this case does well in underscoring the relevance of Shaw's claim that "the greatest problem with communication is the illusion that it has occurred" (George Bernard Shaw as quoted in Hallenbeck et al. 1996, 397).

ADDRESSING LANGUAGE BARRIERS

In the clinical setting, interpreters are vital to helping avoid misunderstandings born out of language differences. They can maximize the amount of information that is conveyed successfully between patients and providers, and increase the number of opportunities to ask and have questions answered. Prima facie, using an interpreter seems like a wonderful idea and a good way to stave off conflict at the outset. Often times this is this case. However, there are several cautionary notes that need to accompany the directive to use an interpreter in the clinical context. It is one thing to request an interpreter for a patient who does not have a friend or family member available to serve as an interpreter. Here it would be difficult to imagine *not* requesting the services of an interpreter. Basic information like symptoms, diagnosis, prognosis, or instructions on how to administer any necessary medications could not be conveyed with any degree of success.

In addition to those who are not able to speak any English, there is a huge population of people that are considered limited in English proficiency (LEP). As of the 2000 U.S. census, approximately "45 million people in the United States speak a language other than English at home, and ~19 million are limited in English proficiency. . . . Five percent of school-aged U.S. children (or ~2.4 million) are LEP, an 85 percent increase since 1979" (Flores et al. 2003, 6). These numbers serve to underscore the importance of having interpreters on hand in the clinical context. Even in the face of clear evidence of their need, interpreters are underutilized.[2] Flores et al. cite one study in which it was found that "no interpreter was used for 46 percent of LEP patients" (Flores et al. 2003, 13). The necessity for interpreter services is apparent in cases where the patient is not able to speak any English. Yet, in cases where a patient is limited in his ability to speak English, but is able to fumble through a basic conversation, there is a danger in overestimating his English speaking capabilities and forgoing the use of an interpreter. The choice not to use an interpreter may be based on several reasons. For instance, in institutions where interpreter services are not easily accessed, obtaining the services of an interpreter may look to be a cumbersome, expensive, time-consuming process. Yet, studies indicate "that trained professional medical interpreter services are associated with improvements in the delivery of health care services to LEP patients, but do not increase the mean duration of medical visits" (Flores 2003, 13). Flores et al. also do well to point out the costs—economic, physical, and psychological—associated with not utilizing a trained professional medical interpreter:

> a successful $71 million lawsuit over a misinterpreted word in the emergency department, a report of a prolonged hospitalization for perforated appendicitis that might have been avoided if an interpreter had been called, and a report of children being placed in state custody for mistaken child abuse because of a misinterpreted word and failure to initially call in an interpreter. (Flores et al. 2003, 13)[3]

These studies buttress the case for offering interpreter services in any case in which differences in language may pose a barrier to communication.[4] These cases would include situations in which patients had friends or family members that spoke some English, but whose language skills would be considered "limited." In such cases, while the intent of offering the services of an interpreter would be to improve communication and decrease the likelihood of misunderstandings and conflict, it might not be seen in this light by everyone involved. As Quill notes, "the use of professional translators when family translators are available can be problematic in many cultures. . . . Inviting an independent translator when family members are available can give a clear message of lack of trust of the family unit" (Quill 2002, 231). This is not to say that using an outside interpreter should be ruled out straight away, but rather, such an invitation should be addressed with the family at the outset in order to explain the rational behind inviting an interpreter to participate in the health care relationship, and to delineate the role of the interpreter. Transparency regarding the intentions and rational behind such decisions is imperative if health care providers are to build trust with their patients. If the interpreter is perceived as threatening, an outsider who may convey important health care information in an incorrect, unflattering light and infringe on an intimate health care provider-patient relationship, then inviting one in may end up doing more harm than good. In their study, Orona et al. note that serious consequences must be noted in opting for a professional interpreter over a family member or friend. Such consequences include, "offending the family when access to the patient/physician dialogue becomes off-limits to them. . . . Questioning the family's veracity and competency, thus leading to a loss of face for the family as well as a loss of rapport between the providers and relatives" (Oronoa et al. 1994, 342). Thus, to go slowly and make it clear that the interpreter is involved only to help the patient or surrogate communicate with the health care provider and vice versa, is an essential first step prior to securing interpreter services. Given the fundamental importance of fostering a foundation of trust, being forthright and inclusive from the first interaction with patient and family is something the importance of which would be hard to overemphasize.

Simply because an outside interpreter is involved it does not follow that there is not an important place for family members in terms of translating for their loved one. This is especially true for discussions surrounding advance care planning, where the issues being discussed are deeply personal. Family members would have a privileged perspective in helping their loved one flesh out a conception of the good life and the values that ought to guide it. Not only would family members be familiar with the patient's history and life narrative, but also they are integral parts of the narrative. This deeply entrenched role for family members, though not unique to any particular group, was manifest in both Chinese and Latino families studied by Orona et al. "The distinctive factor for both Chinese and Latino families in the study was the extent and degree to which extended families became involved in providing care. In addition to their fulfilling their obligation to provide support, relatives also served as reinforcers and validators of the patient's cultural values" (Orona et al. 1994, 341). Often, the questions posed and the responses that are sought in advance care planning are quite nuanced. Family members may be able to convey questions in such a way as to draw out the finer details from the patient, thus obtaining more robust responses. Family members stand in a good position to spark the patient's memory, eliciting rich details that will help others gain a greater understanding of what the patient truly wants when the patient is no longer able to convey such preferences for himself. These finer details may be overlooked if left in the hands of an outside interpreter who is unfamiliar with the patient. To be sure, such details might be left out if an outside interpreter is involved simply because the patient might not feel comfortable discussing such intimate issues with a stranger.

While the potential benefits to be reaped by using a family member or friend as an interpreter are vast, there are weighty reasons in favor of not using someone close to the patient to interpret in the clinical setting. Due to a lack of expertise in the English language, a family member may unintentionally convey information (whether from the patient or physician) incorrectly. Equally as worrisome as these unintentional mistakes, are intentional instances of misinterpretations. Most common amongst intentional mistakes are instances of purposefully miscommunicating the patient's preferences or the physician's recommendations. Intentional miscommunication may stem from a number of different factors. One thing to consider is the potential for a conflict of interest when the interpreter is a friend or family member. For instance, a young man translating for his father might be hard-pressed to be completely forthcoming in delivering a dire prognosis and recommendation to stop further treatments for his father's cancer. The son may want his father to continue to fight so much that he relays a message that the treatments are working and that his father should stay with his current course of treatment. Though born out of good intentions and a love of his father, it is a miscommunication with potentially awful consequences nonetheless.

It might also be the case that the medical information at issue is something that the family member translating is uncomfortable discussing with the patient. For example, it is not hard to imagine how uncomfortable a twenty-year-old grandson would be if charged with the duty of translating for his grandmother at her gynecologist appointment. Because of his discomfort, the grandson may leave out certain questions or comments that he feels would be inappropriate to direct to his grandmother. Numerous other situations in which close family or friends would be uncomfortable translating are not difficult to envisage. More troubling cases in which communication is spoiled intentionally are also not beyond the pale. The following case illustrates an attempt to engage in advance care planning that is thwarted by a family member who willfully misinterprets the expressed wishes of the patient:

Mr. Rodriguez is a seventy-eight-year-old Hispanic man who was diagnosed with lung cancer five years ago. In the past few months his condition has worsened and the cancer has metastasized. He has told his wife that he wants her to be his surrogate and the two of them have come to see his long-time oncologist to draft a living will and durable power of attorney for health care. Mr. Rodriguez speaks very little English, while his wife is quite fluent in it. As such, she agrees to interpret for him, as was always the case during his visits with physicians. Mr. Rodriguez begins by asking his wife to tell the physician that avoiding suffering is of primary importance; it is also paramount that treatments not be initiated if they would only serve to prolong his dying process. In addition, he asked that his wife relay to his physician his preference not to receive artificial nutrition and hydration, in addition to his refusal to be placed on a ventilator for any long-term period (e.g., he was agreeable to the notion of starting him on a ventilator if there was a good chance of weaning him in a few days).

Instead of interpreting as her husband had asked, Mrs. Rodriguez told the physician that her husband had always been a fighter, and that he wanted to maintain that type of character "till the end." Mrs. Rodriguez went on to tell the physician that her husband would want everything possible done to extend his life. The physician explained that given Mr. Rodriguez's poor prognosis and already weakened condition, initiating certain therapies may in fact end up being quite burdensome. Insisting that they were aware of this, Mrs. Rodriguez thanked the physician for the information and checked to make sure that the aggressive treatment preferences she had voiced were documented in her husband's chart. Mr. Rodriguez left the physician's office with a treatment plan that was in stark contrast to the one he actually requested. At his next visit to the oncologist, Mr. Rodriguez had to come without his wife and have one of the Spanish-speaking nurses in the office act as an interpreter. His physician, in trying to clear up a couple of points regarding Mr. Rodriguez's previously documented treatment preferences, was shocked when the nurse relayed a completely different story than Mrs. Rodriguez had just one appointment earlier. Unclear as to which treatment preferences to go with, the oncologist relayed his confusion to Mr. Rodriguez. He then recommended that Mr. Rodriguez go home and speak about this with his wife in order to clear up any uncertainty surrounding such important decisions.

The discussion that ensued between Mr. and Mrs. Rodriguez revealed that the reasons she had for misinterpreting stemmed from a deep concern and love for her husband. To be sure, these beneficent intentions cannot erase the deception and the grave consequences that may have resulted had the situation not been cleared up. Mrs. Rodriguez explained to her husband that she thought he was choosing a less aggressive treatment plan for altruistic reasons—to spare his family the financial and emotional costs that a long, drawn-out end would entail. Mrs. Rodriguez noted that she and her husband were already helping their daughter out both financially and by taking care of her children. Such assistance, though rewarding, was draining in terms of time and money. In light of all of the directions their attention and resources were already being pulled, Mrs. Rodriguez believed that her husband, who had in fact gone through a very aggressive course of treatment when first diagnosed with cancer, was choosing a vastly different plan of care in order to save her from further financial and emotional costs. Confronting her husband directly with these beliefs was not an option, as she thought that it would cause him further distress and possibly serve to dissuade him from doing what he wanted—acting on behalf of his family. That is, his wife thought that Mr. Rodriguez was acting based on the idea common in Hispanic families—that actions ought to be undertaken with a view toward their impact on the family as a whole rather than merely with an eye toward the individual member of the family. Mrs. Rodriguez made it clear to her husband that having him around was what was important, and that if he wanted to go with a more aggressive treatment plan that she would support his decision in full.

In this case, Mr. Rodriguez thought that it was best for his family if he chose a much less aggressive treatment plan. This makes sense in light of the fact that "in most Hispanic families, the needs of the family take precedence over those of the individual" (Galanti 2004, 77). For Mr. Rodriguez, this meant saving his family from an end that would be costly both emotionally and financially, and choosing a much quieter and seemingly quicker end. However, Mr. Rodriguez chose to bear the burden of making this serious decision on his own rather than making it with the whole family. Making such an important decision in isolation runs contrary to common practice in many Hispanic families of familial decision making (Galanti, 2004). Mr. Rodriguez resigned himself to the idea that to include his family in the decision would mean not being able to go with the less aggressive treatment plan that he was sure would be less taxing on his family—the family that would inevitably have to deal with a great loss when he died. He thought that if he were to consult with his family and be transparent about the rationale behind the choice for a less aggressive care plan, that they would convince him to choose otherwise.

Even with the best of intentions, serious complications arose as Mrs. Rodriguez attempted to manipulate the situation by misinterpreting her husband's preferences for care at the end of life. In this case, the physician made a good recommendation when, after recognizing the inconsistencies between what was interpreted by Mrs. Rodriguez compared to the Spanish-speaking nurse, he suggested Mr. and Mrs. Rodriguez discuss treatment preferences openly. Ultimately, Mr. Rodriguez went back to the physician with a care plan that was developed through familial consensus. It was a plan that Mr. Rodriguez was happy with in substance, and also, because he developed it with his family. The plan was a moderate course that combined aspects from the original aggressive treatment plan forwarded by Mrs. Rodriguez, along with components from the much less aggressive treatment plan originally put forth by Mr. Rodriguez. This case serves to highlight the idea that "When treating Hispanic patients, try to involve the family as much as possible. Understand that what affects the one individual affects the entire household" (Galanti 2004, 77). Galanti rightly goes on to note that this statement does not apply uniquely to Hispanic families, but rather, is true of most families regardless of culture. With this in mind, whether dealing with the patient or surrogate directly or through an interpreter, it is a good idea for health care providers to make their *willingness* to include the family in the decision-making process explicit.[5] Overall, this case ended well, but it is easy to imagine an end in which Mr. Rodriguez settled on a care plan that he was not really happy with, where Mrs. Rodriguez never got to make amends for deceiving her husband, and the whole Rodriguez family never got to take part in such a crucial decision-making process.

When it comes to something as personal as advance care planning, several benefits can be gained by having a close family member or friend involved in the process of interpretation. Unfortunately, as was seen in the Rodriguez case, there are also potential drawbacks that can be quite serious that come with having someone in whom the patient has complete trust do the interpreting. When involving family members or friends in the interpretation process, a good rule of thumb is to be vigilant about any conflicting statements.[6] That is, do the statements made by the family-member-interpreter seem to go against the preferences voiced by the patient (possibly through an interpreter) in the past? In other words, are the present preferences ones that could be considered part of a coherent whole? If the answer is yes, then while the provider must still remain vigilant for clues that the patient's voice is being stifled in some way, coherence should offer the provider some solace in that the current preferences are not anomalous. However, while having a coherent, consistent set of preferences may offer some comfort to the provider that the interpreter is "getting it right," if the most current preferences are vastly different than those expressed in the past, it does not necessarily follow that the interpreter is, for whatever reason, misinterpreting what the patient is saying. It could simply be the case that circumstances have changed, moving the patient to change his mind regarding a plan of care. Thus, lack of coherence is cause for further probing, not automatic incredulity and suspicion of the interpreter. When the interpreter being used is a close friend or family member of the patient, the health care provider must make sure that preferences of the patient are being translated correctly. A good way to do this is to establish a relationship with the patient based on trust and openness, focusing on keeping the lines of communication clear. In advance care planning, where the treatments at issue determine how a person will spend the last days of his life, ensuring that patient preferences are translated accurately and everyone involved feels comfortable asking questions is of paramount importance.[7]

A ROBUST CONCEPTION OF THE ROLE OF MEDICAL INTERPRETERS IN ADVANCE CARE PLANNING

In terms of identifying and facing some of the obstacles that arise in attempting to engage in advance care planning across cultures, medical interpreters can provide valuable insight. One area where interpreters have noted a potential for confusion is in the different approaches health care providers and patients may take in asking and answering questions. Specifically, is there an expectation for a direct and explicit question-and-answer exchange? Or rather, is the norm a more circuitous conversation in which questions are not always posed as directly as they could be, and answers may come (if at all) only after the question is asked several times (in several different ways)? One interpreter explained the problem in the following way:

> When you ask [patients] a question, they're going to respond to another, unrelated question. And the doctors, well they have to keep a schedule, they're not

there to repeat the same question 5 times in a row. They get angry. But in our country, this is very common. The questions are never direct. . . . But the doctor thinks that the interpreter isn't doing his job. (Hudelson 2005, 314)

Misalignment in either style and/or expectation of communication can be disastrous in terms of engaging in advance care planning. To begin with, advance care planning is not and should not be expected to be a speedy endeavor. The issues common to advance care planning are often those that are broached infrequently. They are usually deeply personal and are commonly those things that "go unsaid"—even between close friends and family members. It is a difficult task to articulate responses to complicated questions like "What makes life worth living?" "What makes life valuable?" "What would an 'unacceptable' life look like?" Such questions are intrinsically difficult to answer. Any expectation that they might be addressed quickly must be dismissed. Instead, careful attention and devoted time must be given to this delicate process.

Another concern that may influence the success (or lack thereof) of the advance care planning process is the potential for patients not familiar with Western medicine to be unclear about what are taken in Western medicine to be fundamental concepts. During the advance care planning process, it is not uncommon to discuss the types of conditions that one would deem unacceptable in terms of quality of life. In discussing such conditions, the idea of being dependent upon various medications and/or machines for medical treatment will likely be broached. Yet, the concept of having to be hooked up to a machine at all, let alone for any extended period of time, may be something of which an individual has never conceived. To be sure, one may not be familiar with the idea of taking medications for longer than a few days at most. It may be the case in some cultures that treating sick individuals is more of an acute event in which "treatment" is given to the individual and then, perhaps, prayers or blessings are said on behalf of the sick individual for some extended time period. In such cases, "treatment plans" might be more aptly referred to as "prayer plans." As Chesanow explains, "Taking medications over an extended period for a chronic condition, may be unknown concepts in the patient's culture" (Chesanow 1998, 146). For example, if one's condition necessitates going for dialysis several times a week along with several other medical treatments, the profound impact that such a course will have on a person's life is difficult to convey to someone who is unfamiliar with chronic care. Medical interpreters can work to bridge the gap in communication, breaking down complex concepts into more "digestible," simpler parts. In addition, medical interpreters can also focus on controlling the pace at which difficult information is conveyed. Here interpreters could focus on making sure that complex concepts are not simply glossed over too quickly. Because of the weight of preferences documented in an advance directive, health care providers need to be aware of the disparities in terms of starting points between patient and provider. That is, when even fundamental concepts are not shared, extreme caution must be taken in explaining and guiding the advance care planning process. Paying close attention to nonverbal cues along with setting aside ample time for questions and explanations regarding the various aspects of the advance care planning process are but a few of the things medical interpreters can help highlight the importance of in order to facilitate the advance care planning process in a multicultural clinical setting.

BODY LANGUAGE: WHAT'S IN A NOD?

When practicing in a multicultural setting, it becomes clear that even the seemingly most benign assumptions can serve to create conflict and discord. Such dangers were apparent when discussing language differences and the use of interpreters. As important as what a patient says while interacting with health care providers is the patient's body language. Just as with verbal communication, assumptions can prove hazardous when it comes to body language. For instance, in some cultures making eye contact is a way of signaling that one is paying attention to what the speaker is saying and doing. It is a sign that one is engaged in the discussion. Some may even take eye contact as a sign of self-confidence, possibly even as a sign that the individual is being honest and forthright (e.g., "he looked me straight in the eye"). Conversely, *avoiding* eye contact in some cultures is taken as a sign of concern and caring. For example, there is a Navaho belief that "the eyes are the windows to the soul. To make direct eye contact is disrespectful and can endanger the spirits of both parties" (Galanti 2004, 33). Avoiding eye contact in the Navaho culture can therefore be understood as a way for individuals to look out for each other.

While eye contact is usually interpreted as a sign of respect, honesty, and self-confidence in a Western culture, it may be seen as disrespectful in many Asian cultures. Given the hierarchical nature of some cultures, those in a "lower" or "subordinate" position are taught not to look their "superiors" in the eye—to do so would be to imply (incorrectly) that they are "equals" (Galanti 2004, 34). Whether eye contact is perceived as a sign of respect or a means by which to show disrespect, whether it indicates honesty or a "sexual invitation,"[8] the one thing to note about eye contact (or lack thereof) regardless of the cultural groups at play, is that the only way to really know why someone does or does not make eye contact is to ask him. Having an awareness of the fact that eye contact can convey a number of different things helps providers to realize how careful and proactive they need to be in making sure that a common understanding of the situation is achieved.

Confusion can also arise when it comes to the simple gesture of nodding one's head. Taken by many cultures (e.g., Euro-American) to signify agreement or understanding, nodding one's head in some Latin American and Asian cultures can convey very different meanings. Crawley et al. discuss a case in which Mrs. Martinez, a Spanish-speaking sixty-seven-year-old immigrant from El Salvador living in the United States with her daughter, is asked by her physician about her preferences for treatment at the end of life (Crawley et al. 2002, 674). Since her daughter was not at the clinic visit with her mother, the physician asked that a trained medical interpreter be present. After the discussion, the interpreter tells the physician that Mrs. Martinez is confused about several issues including why she, rather than her family, was being asked to make such decisions, and whether there would be any legal repercussions regarding her immigration status if she signed any of the forms from her health care provider. Such confusion existed even though during the interpreter-facilitated conversation Mrs. Martinez continued to nod her head. Mrs. Martinez's physician took such nodding as a sign of understanding and "assent." The interpreter also, "suggests that Mrs. Martinez's nodding indicates politeness and respect for the physician, not assent" (Crawley et al. 2002, 674). Had the interpreter not suggested this alternate interpretation of a head nod, the physician may have remained under the impression that Mrs. Martinez understood and was in agreement with what had been proposed by the physician. Even more, during future visits the physician may have remained under the impression that a head nod meant understanding and agreement and not pursued things further or made sure to probe Mrs. Martinez to see if she had any questions that she was reticent to ask.

Overall, when dealing with patients from different cultures, health care providers need not be aware of all of the nuances of every gesture in every culture. Clearly that is an impossible goal. What is imperative for health care providers to do is to be aware of the fact that various gestures may mean different things in different cultures. For example, there can be great variations in the amount of distance that people should maintain between one another, questions regarding whether or not touching is permissible beyond what is necessary for physical examination, all the way to what might be meant by particular gestures. "Some cultures consider finger pointing or foot pointing disrespectful (Asian), while others consider vigorous handshaking a sign of aggression (Native American) or a gesture of good will (European American)" (Trotter, accessed July 16, 2008). Simply acknowledging the potential that different meanings might be conveyed by the same gesture is a necessary first step in diminishing the likelihood of misunderstanding and conflict in a pluralistic setting.

NOTES

1. Italics are mine.
2. The need for interpreters was supported in deed when,

In August 2000, the federal Office for Civil Rights (OCR) of the Department of Health and Human Services mandated that any entities that receive federal funds, including health care organizations (e.g., through Medicaid or the Children's Health Insurance Program), "must offer and provide language assistance services, including bilingual staff and interpreter services, at no cost to each patient/consumer with limited English proficiency at all points of contact, in a timely manner during all hours of operation." This is not a new law, but rather a clarification of Title VI of the Civil Rights Act of 1964. Essentially, service providers who fail to provide meaningful access to individuals with LEP are considered to be discriminating based on national origin. (www.accessproject.org/ downloads/c_LEPEngembarg.pdf, accessed August 22, 2007)

3. A report on WebMD highlighted the economic sense it makes to utilize medical interpreters:

In 1997, emergency medicine specialist Louis Hampers compared the care given to patients at a Chicago hospital who were not fluent in English to the care given those who were. Non-English speakers tended to be admitted to the hospital more often and they were given more IV fluids and unnecessary tests. Hampers . . . tells WebMD that addressing the language barrier in health care not only makes sense from an ethical standpoint, but from a legal and business standpoint as well. "If you can prevent one hospitalization for every 100 patients by having an interpreter, that interpreter would no doubt pay for themselves." (www.webmd.com/news/20060719/language-barrier-affecting-health-care, accessed August 8, 2007)

4. To be sure, it may seem that medicine has a language accessible only to health care providers. On this presupposition, interpreters would be needed for most clinical encounters. Thus, when I refer to differences in language that pose barriers to patient-provider communication, I am referring to situations in which individuals with limited English proficiency are seeking care in an English-speaking clinical context.

5. Such a willingness on the part of the providers is constrained by the patient's preferences regarding how much or how little additional family members are to be involved in the decision-making process. The point here is that the opportunity to involve the family in the decision-making process should not be impeded by the unwillingness of a health care provider to accommodate such a request.

6. The following is a recommendation from the U.S. Department of Health and Human Services, National Standards for Culturally and Linguistically Appropriate Services in Health Care:

In order to ensure complete, accurate, impartial, and confidential communication, family, friends or other individuals, should not be required, suggested, or used as interpreters. A patient/consumer may choose to use a family member or friend as an interpreter after being informed of the availability of free interpreter services unless the effectiveness of services is compromised or the LEP person's confidentiality is violated. The health care organization's staff should suggest that a trained interpreter be present during the encounter to ensure accurate interpretation and should document the offer and declination in the LEP person's file. Minor children should never be used as interpreters, nor be allowed to interpret for their parents when they are the patients/consumers. (2001, 12)

While this recommendation is well-founded, the ability to heed it may tend to vary on the resources available to the institution at issue, as well as other demographic factors. This recommendation underscores the need for vigilance when involving close friends and family members; parties with interests deeply vested in the outcome of the interpreting process. At the same time, it leaves room for such parties because it recognizes the value that they can add to the process.

7. Chapter 5 will focus on specific tools available to help health care providers facilitate communication with patients and surrogates.

8. As Galanti notes, "Many Middle Easterners regard direct eye contact between a man and a woman as a sexual invitation. . . . In general, eye contact should be avoided with Middle Easterners of the opposite sex" (Galanti 2004, 35).

Chapter Four

Truth-Telling and Disclosure

It is tranquility and serenity a sick person needs, not knowledge.

—Gordon and Paci (1997, 1439)

DISCLOSURE: TITRATING THE TRUTH

Determining what information is conveyed to the patient is as important as ensuring that information is communicated clearly and accurately, and in a culturally sensitive manner. Dating back to Hippocrates, physicians were cautioned "to [conceal] most things from the patient while attending to him; [to] give necessary orders with cheerfulness and serenity . . . revealing nothing of the patient's future or present condition" (Hippocrates, as cited in Arras and Steinbock 1998, 87). Such a practice lies in stark contrast to the current practice in Western medicine of including the patient, as much as possible, in the medical decision-making process. Emphasis on open, free-flowing lines of communication between patient and provider is founded on the "dominant, middle-class, European-American ethos, [in which] the individual is viewed as autonomous, egalitarian, rational, self-assertive, and self-aware. Cultivation of the rational mind is of the essence, and healthy interpersonal relationships are characterized by open, verbal communication" (Kawaga-Singer and Kassim-Lakha 2003, 580). On this model, the individual's input is weighted heavily, and is meaningful only insofar as it is informed. Health care providers are the ones with the medical knowledge and expertise necessary to inform the patient's decision. As such, they are in the best position not just to treat the patient's condition, but also, to educate the patient about his condition so that he can determine and decide on the treatment option that aligns

59

with his values and preferences. Thus, a complete picture of a good health care provider is one who tends not only to the patient's ailment, but also to the patient as a person. The former is a function of being a good practitioner of medicine, the latter is a much harder skill to acquire—one which comes only when one learns how to listen well and is willing and able to keep an open mind. Mastering the skills of a good practitioner will, ideally, lead to better outcomes in terms of greater patient satisfaction and less conflict overall between patients and health care providers.

While communication that is open and forthright is often prized in the Western biomedical model, this style of communication is not universally accepted. There are some cultures in which the relaying of a poor prognosis to the patient directly, without even consulting the family, is an act that may be construed as an insult, and possibly even a cruel and serious harm. The notion that providing information to the patient about the patient's condition could amount to a (grave) harm stands in direct opposition to a standard Western, biomedical perspective in which a lack of full disclosure would be perceived as disrespectful and a harm.[1] The multicultural nature of the health care landscape has made it necessary for providers to recognize that there are numerous conceptions of what proper disclosure ought to look like. Finding a balance when faced with differing conceptions, determining what information to disclose in terms of both substance and quantity, is a difficult skill to develop but one that is a necessary component in the repertoire of a good health care provider.

Several reasons are cited as driving the request for less-than-full disclosure. For instance, the concept of protection is common to discussions of disclosure in the medical setting. Often, relatives of patients who request that medical information be withheld from the patient maintain that part of their role as a family member is to protect their loved one from negative health information. As Beyene explains, "For Ethiopians, 'bad news' should be told to a family member or close friend of the patient at appropriate times and places and in a culturally approved and recognized manner" (Beyene 1992, 328). Ethiopians think that it is not the proper place of the doctor, who is usually not as close to the patient as a friend or family member, to be the one to deliver "bad news." Friends and family members will be in the best position to relay the information to the patient, in the manner most appropriate for the patient. Relatives see themselves as shielding the patient from the harsh reality of a poor medical prognosis. This is especially true when the ill family member is elderly. This need to protect ill family members runs deep, instantiating itself as a duty that is taken very seriously. Orona et al. found this "duty to protect" common to both the Chinese and Latino families involved in their study. "Duty" was defined by both Latino and Chinese relatives as protecting the patient (typically an elderly parent) by making the remaining time comfortable and free of distress. Central to protection was a need to keep information about the disease and prognosis from the patient (Orona et al. 1994, 341). Chinese relatives rooted this duty in their "Confucianist tradition," while Latino families had a general recognition of such a duty as part of and integral to their "cultural identity" (Orona et al. 1994).

In Japan, where advance directives have no formal legal standing, various organizations have developed documents that serve as informal vehicles used to document patient preferences. While these documents are not legally binding, they have varying degrees of influence depending upon the individual practitioner at issue (Kimura 1998). The Citizen's Group in Thinking of Terminal Care issued one such document "which attempted to simplify matters by providing a place for a check mark in front of each statement. . . . Sentence No. 1 says, 'please tell to my family members as it is but don't tell me the truth clearly'" (Kimura 1998). Given the explicit mention of and prominent position granted to the preference not to be (at least) "fully informed," one is able to see that such a preference is not uncommon in Japanese culture.

Across various cultures, at the core of this duty to protect was the idea that receiving too much information can be harmful to the patient. For example, "harm" could be done by disclosing the truth about a poor prognosis to a patient, thus causing the patient to lose hope. To be sure, an individual would probably know that she is ill, and even further, would likely know when the illness seems to be getting worse. Nonetheless, it is one thing to suspect that you are not doing well, it is something else entirely to be told explicitly that your illness is terminal and that you have only a few months (if that) to live. Disclosure of such information is tremendously difficult to take no matter what your culture. Even for those who prize honesty and forthrightness, such a prognosis would be a tough blow. Compound the difficulty of hearing such news with a view that frowns upon disclosing such information to the patient directly, and you have, at best, a brutal strike to an individual and her conception of how illness is handled. Latino patients in one study viewed the practice of full disclosure as "destroying all hope for the terminally ill person . . . once a diagnosis is made of a terminal illness with an 'end point,' hope is destroyed" (Orona et al. 1994, 339). While there is an anxiety tied to living in uncertainty, there still exists alongside it a niche for hope. Once someone is told that his condition is terminal, hope is, at least, greatly diminished. According to Chan, one of the main reasons why the family and not the patient is told that the patient is terminally ill is because telling the patient this information would "undermine the normal relations among family members, because they could not act as if nothing had happened once the truth was disclosed" (Chan 2004, 94).

Conversely, on the biomedical model, while hope might be diminished in light of being given a poor prognosis, such information also provides the patient with an opportunity. Specifically, it allows an individual to make important health care decisions that are more fully informed. An individual is thus provided with the materials necessary to utilize her rational capacities to determine what her treatment plan will look like. It will allow her to reign in some control and be an active participant in her own health care. In addition, providing such information to the patient would also help to paint an accurate picture of the severity of the situation, taking away any *false* hope that may have developed. In contrast, if you are from a culture where such unabashed forthrightness is viewed with disdain, where patient participation in treatment at the end of life is unheard of, disclosure represents an affront to the individual, an act of cruelty tantamount to extinguishing all hope:

> In Italy, cultural meanings of cancer as a disease and of disclosure are framed within the value of providing hope to the patient. An underlying cultural value holds that one must spare the suffering of others, where having full disclosure disrupts the "serenity" of the terminally ill cancer patient. (Orona et al. 1994, 339)

To be sure, the value placed on maintaining hope is so high that to take away hope from a sick individual is tantamount to relegating him to a life not worth living. Hope is seen as a glue that holds families together and allows for them to continue on: it is a source of strength; to take hope away is to commit one to a kind of death, "Finché c'è vita, c'èsperanza"[2] (Gordon and Paci 1997, 1444).

Along the same line, some people may subscribe to the idea that one role of a patient's family is to take on the burden of worry and stress for the patient. Given that the patient is already compromised by her illness, she should be spared the encumbrance of worry and anxiety that comes along with all of the details of the diagnosis and prognosis. Feeling better, concentrating on getting well and staying positive are the tasks of the patient. Handling all of the negative information and the stress that comes along with it is a burden for family members to bear. In fact, such a practice does not seem to be quite so far from the practices commonly found on a Western model.[3] Family members often "pick up the slack" for a sick relative. This may include helping out more with the upkeep of a house, to caring for children, to something altogether different. What is common though, is the notion that family members often take on such roles because they believe it to be their duty to do so. Thus, the concept of "filial duty," though expressed in different ways and in varying degrees, is something that cuts across cultures. Overall, understanding the role of the family in caring for a loved one is crucial to understanding how disclosure is viewed. For instance, in many cultures primacy is given to concerns about the family as a whole as opposed to concerns about any particular individual member of the family. In a study measuring attitudes toward end-of-life decision making with Japanese and Japanese-American[4] focus groups, there was agreement across all groups that familial concerns were more important than personal concerns—even those concerns regarding personal suffering (Bito et al. 2007). In describing what a "good death" would look like, participants in all groups emphasized not wanting to be a burden to others. Ideally, death would not be prolonged, but rather, one would die suddenly "*pokkuri*" or "popping off" (Bito et al. 2007, 255). Further,

> nearly all participants expressed negative feelings toward living in adverse health states. Nonetheless, they focused minimally on personal suffering. Instead, participants focused on the level of caregiving burden that would be borne by their families, and all groups expressed a strong unwillingness to burden others. (Bito et al. 2007, 255)

Disclosing information to the family allows family members to discharge their duty to protect and care for their loved one. If important information is kept from them they might be hindered in this endeavor. If troubling information is given to the patient directly, the patient might lose hope and withdraw from life. If that happens, family members might feel as though they failed in their obligations. Resting control in the hands of the family is seen as a way to ensure that patients are protected and family members can fulfill their obligations.

The duty to protect the patient is not exclusive to the family. Such a role also falls under the purview of health care providers. At first blush it may not seem very difficult for a health care provider to serve as an additional "protector" of her patient. However, discharging this duty is complicated by several factors, not the least of which is the very call that is fundamental to this book—the call to increase cultural sensitivity. While it is clear that there is a dearth of cultural sensitivity in health care, overcompensating by becoming absolutely deferential to the expressed cultural dictates of others is a practice that is rife with danger. Brotzman and Butler illustrate this danger in the following case of a fifty-eight-year-old Hmong woman diagnosed with incurable pancreatic cancer:

> The woman did not speak any English, and her family would not tell her the diagnosis. Nine months after the patient's disease was diagnosed, her oldest son told physicians that such information is not given to the dying in the Hmong culture because it is believed to hasten the patient's death. This was confirmed when the concerned physician, faced with increasingly frequent questions from the patient about her growing discomfort, asked advice from Southeast Asian and other health care providers. . . . The physician pressed the matter with the

family . . . gaining from them the admission that they did not adhere to this
particular belief, but were reluctant to tell the patient her poor prognosis for
other reasons . . . mainly on the fear that the patient would become depressed
and they would be unable to help her. After discussion, the family did reveal
the patient's prognosis to her, and, following an adjustment period, the woman
began to prepare for her death. (1991, 426)

This case serves as a nice example of why health care providers need to
engage families in discussions in an attempt to glean the rationale behind treatment requests that they may make. One ought not accept blindly nor take as a
sufficient condition for action, the reason "it is a cultural mandate." The physician in this case did well not to accept the family's reasoning for withholding
the truth from the patient at face value. While it did take the physician nine
months to tease out this information from the family,[5] the actual reason why the
family was requesting that the patient not be told of her diagnosis was eventually revealed. The physician should be commended for consulting broadly,
taking advantage of human resources—Southeast Asian and other health care
providers in the area—who offer a privileged perspective. Such "resources" are
often overlooked. Striking this balance between appreciating and accommodating the cultural preferences and practices of patients, and discharging the duty
as a health care provider to protect your patient is not easy. Providers trained
within the biomedical model would be working off of the presupposition that
it is their charge to provide information to the patient in an effort to further the
principles of veracity and patient autonomy, while at the same time being faced
with the realization that the very information they seem obligated to disclose
may in fact violate the principles of beneficence and nonmaleficence.

In order to determine how to proceed, a health care provider must be aware
of a few things. First, she needs to be clear on the reasoning behind the request
for nondisclosure. To not disclose information about diagnosis and prognosis to
the patient stands in opposition to standard practice on the biomedical model.
Thus, to act contrary to this standard requires a solid justification. Further, as
was seen in the case above, even when reasons are given, they need not be
taken at face value. Though it may be difficult, the health care provider, when
in doubt, may need to probe to see how accurately the rationale given aligns
with the true beliefs and values of the patient and family. To be sure, it will be
a rare family that would not be acting with a beneficent intent, and who would
not be in the best position to convey, in an appropriate manner and amount,
information to the patient. But, in an effort to uphold a moral requirement of
the biomedical model—disclosing the diagnosis and prognosis to the patient
and soliciting patient involvement in development of a treatment plan—health
care practitioners need to remain vigilant. Ultimately, the culturally sensitive

provider will be the one who, with an eye toward the practice of disclosure found in the biomedical model, tries to incorporate the cultural beliefs of her patients to the greatest degree possible. It is this focus on understanding and integrating the cultural beliefs of patients into the medical decision-making process and development of the medical treatment plan that is crucial to providing health care in a culturally sensitive manner. As can be gathered from above, the practice of full disclosure foundational in the biomedical model is not necessarily the "right" way, and certainly not the only way to engage with patients and families. For instance,

> From inside the non-disclosing perspective of some Italians, the "American approach" looks very harsh, irresponsible, lonely, naïve. It looks as if, at the time the patient needs to rest, be cared for and protected by others, s/he has tremendous responsibility and work to do: understand the diagnosis and prognosis, decide on what therapy to follow, work at therapy, have a positive attitude, express deep and strong emotions and thoughts, and plan "rationally" for one's future end. Knowing looks very courageous or foolish or dangerous, and seems the cause of unnecessary suffering. (Gordon and Paci 1997, 1448)

For a culturally sensitive provider, the cultural beliefs and practices of her patient are an integral part of providing quality health care. Making an exerted effort to respect them must be a priority in caring for patients in a multicultural setting.

DOCUMENTING PREFERENCES:
A REQUIREMENT FOR SOME, A DISHONOR FOR OTHERS

The guiding norm in Western medicine is for the health care provider to document patient preferences in the chart or medical record. To be sure, such a practice is not the standard in and only in Western medicine. Documentation is important for many reasons. First, health care teams in hospitals are vastly different than those of the not-so-distant past in which a "standard" care team consisted of one physician and a couple of nurses. At present, it is rare that during a stay in hospital an individual would be seen by only one physician representing one specialty. Health care teams today usually consist of several different people, representing various professions including, but not limited to, medicine, nursing, social work, pharmacy, speech pathology, respiratory therapy, and nutrition. These various roles are filled by different individuals, rotating in and out of cases on a daily basis. The medical chart is a tool with which members of the health care team communicate with one another. For many, it is the sole means by which communication with some members of the team occurs. Important information like patient preferences regarding treatment, and even the values that underlie such preferences should be noted in the chart for all of the members of the team to be aware of and by which to be guided. Documenting patient preferences provides members of the health care team with a point of reference. Intermittently, health care providers should revisit the noted preferences. This way, team members can ensure that they are familiar with the patient preferences, that such preferences have not changed, and if they have changed, note the proper amendments.

While the reasons to document patient preferences are overwhelming, the issue of documentation is not without complexity. The following case serves to point out some of the issues that should be addressed when doing something as routine as documenting the preferences and corresponding rationales for patient treatment choices:

Mr. Kahleed is a fifty-eight-year-old Jordanian man with congestive heart failure. Recently, his condition has worsened quite a bit. He is constantly short of breath and the swelling in his legs has gotten so bad that he needs a wheelchair to get around outside of the home. At a scheduled visit to the cardiologist, Mr. Kahleed laments that he is no longer enjoying his life. He explains to his physician, Dr. Riley, that he is unable to work, engage in any activity that involves more than minimal exertion, and is generally uncomfortable most of the day. He asks Dr. Riley if any treatment options are available that might help him "get more out of his daily life." Given Dr. Riley's long-standing relationship with Mr. Kahleed, coupled with a relatively clear picture of the course his illness would take, Dr. Riley was able to draw out helpful details in terms of Mr. Kahleed's preferences. Dr. Riley explained that the options were limited at best, and that Mr. Kahleed's prognosis was not good. Dr. Riley then attempted to begin a dialogue to determine how aggressive a treatment plan Mr. Kahleed would prefer in light of his deteriorating health. Ultimately, it became clear that Mr. Kahleed preferred a treatment plan that would allow for aggressive treatment only insofar as such treatment might restore him to a baseline where he can enjoy some of the things he determined made his life worth living—eating meals with his family, living at home (as opposed to in some type of health care facility), and being able to play card games. Dr. Riley agreed to fashion a care plan in light of this information, and then proceeded to write down the main points from his conversation with Mr. Kahleed, checking to make sure that they were in agreement in terms of a care plan. Mr. Kahleed told Dr. Riley that his wife would be the one to look to for medical decision making if he should become incompetent. Dr. Riley then proceeded to ask Mr. Kahleed to write down his wishes in his own words, to make sure that Mr. Kahleed's preferences were noted as accurately as possible. In addition, Dr. Riley made a further suggestion that Mr. Kahleed formally appoint his wife (with whom Mr. Kahleed consulted on medical matters) to be his surrogate. This way, if differences arose in choosing treatment options for Mr. Kahleed, his wife would have a formal surrogate designation and be in a stronger position (legally speaking) to direct her husband's treatment plan. Dr. Riley asked that Mr. Kahleed bring the signed paperwork back to the office so that it could be placed in the medical record. Mr. Kahleed became quite upset at this suggestion and proceeded to leave the office, visibly angered.

From Dr. Riley's perspective, Mr. Kahleed's behavior is perplexing at best. It would seem as though Dr. Riley had done nothing wrong. Patient autonomy was given primacy and actions were taken to ensure that the patient's values drove the decision-making process. On this view, Dr. Riley acted responsibly, trying to make sure that Mr. Kahleed's treatment plan was in line with his expressed preferences and relayed by a surrogate of his choosing—his wife. However, Mr. Kahleed viewed Dr. Riley's actions through a very different lens, shaped by his Jordanian background. Specifically, Mr. Kahleed took issue with the fact that Dr. Riley asked him to put his preferences in writing, and also to have documentation drawn up that would formally appoint his wife to be his surrogate if he became incompetent. Werth et al. explain that, "for some Arab Americans, a verbal agreement is more important than a written one, and not accepting a verbal contract may imply that one does not trust the person and therefore one is dishonoring the patient" (Werth et al. 2002, 208). For Dr. Riley to ask for Mr. Kahleed to put his wishes in writing was tantamount to saying that he did not trust his word.

In light of this incident, trust needed to be rebuilt and misunderstandings clarified. At Mr. Kahleed's next appointment Dr. Riley begins by sitting down and asking what had caused Mr. Kahleed to get so upset at his last appointment (a question Dr. Riley was not able to get out before Mr. Kahleed stormed out of the office during his last appointment). Mr. Kahleed, who has always liked Dr. Riley, explains that in his culture verbal agreements are quite weighty. A person's word carries at least as much force as would a written contract from a Western perspective. Hence, when Mr. Kahleed engaged in an in-depth conversation regarding his treatment and surrogate preferences with Dr. Riley, he thought that would have been sufficient to ensure, as much as possible, that his wishes would be followed. Dr. Riley's request that Mr. Kahleed put his preferences in writing was perceived as an even greater blow, since he had just engaged in a deeply personal dialogue with a physician he thought he could trust and one that he believed trusted him.

Dr. Riley explained to Mr. Kahleed that having his preferences in writing would help to make sure that his wishes were followed. Far from intending to offend him, Dr. Riley explained that he made the request out of a concern for doing everything he could to make sure the last chapter of Mr. Kahleed's life was directed by Mr. Kahleed. Further, having his preferences in writing would also help to make sure that caregivers other than Dr. Riley would know what Mr. Kahleed wanted. Dr. Riley also explained that by having Mr. Kahleed's preferences documented in the chart (and potentially in a formal advance directive), caregivers would be able to have a reference point from which to work. Specifically, as different treatment options arise, caregivers would be able to discuss them in light of Mr. Kahleed's noted values and preferences. To be sure, by revisiting them intermittently, the health care team would be able to determine whether Mr. Kahleed's preferences had changed, and amend them as appropriate.

Placing a large amount of stock in the spoken word and verbal agreements is not unique to someone with a Jordanian lineage. As Chan explains, in Japan "verbal instruction is regarded as an adequate means of communication in a harmonious family. It is inappropriate to articulate one's wishes in writing, as this would be perceived as a sign of not trusting other family members" (Chan 2004, 94). In the same vein, Kimura notes that the gravity of the issues typically addressed in advance directives ought not be dealt with in a written document,[6] but rather in a "more harmonious way," a sort of "tacit agreement" (or "Ishin-denshin"—"heart to heart communication without words") between the parties involved the decision-making process (Kimura 1998). The issues dealt with in advance directives are not seen as the stuff of written documents developed for legal purposes. Instead, such topics are to be discussed between individuals who, in conjunction with the health care team, decide what to do for the patient based on a deep love for and knowledge of the patient within the context of his family.

Ultimately, what could have been done to help avoid this misunderstanding? A good way for health care providers to approach sensitive issues, regardless of whether they share the same cultural background as the patient, is to make sure to provide a bit of an explanation when making requests or recommending a particular course of action. For instance, prior to requesting that Mr. Kahleed put his preferences in writing, Dr. Riley could have talked a bit about the importance of even discussing the issues involved in planning for care at the end of life. With that said, he could go on to explain that putting such wishes in writing will help make sure that they are followed. Even more, it is helpful to note, when appropriate, that certain requests or recommendations are asked as a matter of course. This will help to make it clear that the patient is not being singled out, but rather, that the request or practice is routine—that to not ask would be out of the norm. Making the patient feel as though he has been singled out may serve to isolate him and create distance between patient and provider. Offering the patient insight into why requests are made and courses of action recommended will help put the patient at ease and foster trust upon which to build a strong patient-provider relationship. With such a solid foundation off of which to work, progress will be easier to achieve in delving into highly personal matters like those common in advance care planning.

DISCLOSURE AND ADVANCE CARE PLANNING

How one views disclosure, both in terms of what it will look like and whether or not it should even occur, directly influences the advance care planning process. This is especially true in cases where the individual has been diagnosed with a terminal illness or has been dealing with a chronic illness, the course of which is not completely foreign. What is special about this predicament is that one could be fairly specific regarding preferences and values in light of certain expected or predictable complications associated with the disease. This allows a bit more specificity and detail during the advance care planning process—a process that is often criticized for its ambiguity. Given this insight, this privileged perspective, a patient in such circumstances would be a prime candidate for engaging in advance care planning. In cultures where the patient is not told that he is terminally ill, he would be robbed of the opportunity to imbue his wishes, via an advance directive,[7] into the medical decision-making process should he become incompetent. To be sure, lack of disclosure (or at least full disclosure) might be seen by some as standard practice—something that is not only accepted, but is required. In such cases, the patient would not feel robbed of any opportunities. What is essential in either case is making sure that the patient is amenable to the idea of not receiving such information and not having the opportunity to explicitly state the values he would want guiding his treatment plan in case of incompetence.

Similarly, in cases where disclosure is not the norm, advance care planning might be seen as irrelevant. That is, when an individual becomes ill, decisions regarding medical treatment fall under the purview of the family, not the patient. The patient would not be involved in such planning, but rather, would be focused on getting well. To a patient in such circumstances, engaging in advance care planning would be at best a waste of time and energy. In addition, advance care planning might be seen as a waste of time because of the lack of weight placed on any advance directive that might develop out of such a process. As Chan points out, in Japan, "the decision of an individual, even stated in a living will, can be overridden by the collective decision of a family" (Chan 2004, 94). Thus, even if one goes through the advance care planning process and drafts an advance directive (here specifically a living will), primacy will be given to the collective decision of the family and not, as is common in the biomedical model,[8] the decision of the patient as stated in the advance directive. To undertake the task of developing an advance directive, knowing that there is a chance that it can, and very well may, be overridden, might seem to be a waste of time and energy. Expending such resources in light of how easily the directive can be overturned could easily be seen as more of a burden than a benefit to an individual already taxed by illness.

Advance directives, in Japanese cultures for instance, may not be very appealing due to a difference in the way one understands oneself in relation to others. For example, in Japan it is traditional to understand oneself with a sense of "interdependence," "*Amae*," as part of a larger whole and in relationship with others (Kimura 1998). Given a culture in which individuals understand themselves to be part of a much larger whole, it stands to reason that drafting an advance directive—a document that stands as a paradigm manifestation of individual autonomy—would not be a priority. In such cases, autonomy would be not be seen as "empowering," but instead would be "perceived as isolating and burdensome" (Zimring 2001, 242). The decisions typical to advance directives are simply not understood as those that would fall under the discretion of the individual. Rather, they would be made by the family as a whole with input, ranging in amount and weightiness, from various members. The authority granted to the family is not understood as an attempt to usurp power from the individual. Indeed, such authority never rested in the hands of the individual—it was always embedded within the fabric of the family as a whole. Candib, drawing on her earlier work (Candib 1995) and the work of Fan (1997) and Gostin (1995) describes this familial take on autonomy as follows:

> We can move from an individualistic notion of autonomy in healthcare— which concerns itself with protecting individuals from power abuses and paternalism of the medical care system—to a family-based autonomy that protects "persons-in-relation" from the isolation and alienation of the sick within the medical care system. Decision-making will flow not from one's separateness as an individual but from one's connectedness as a family member. (Candib 2002, 225)

Health care providers need to be aware of this conception of autonomy, a conception that seems to deviate so dramatically from the picture of the individual as self-governing and authoritative in the decision-making process, in order to understand and communicate effectively with patients who understand autonomy in this way.

RETHINKING THE FOCUS OF ADVANCE CARE PLANNING

Even when advance directives are viewed as having little weight, and/or when family members are charged with the task of making medical decisions, there is a case to be made for engaging in advance care planning. Advance care planning would focus, for instance, on supporting the patient's preference to have family members make decisions for him in case he became incompetent. Unfortunately, when an individual becomes incompetent there are no guarantees that the people the patient wants to be making health care decisions will in fact be the ones at the helm. Thus, the importance of formally designating individuals to take on the role of surrogate would be underscored. In other words, formally appointing someone to take on the role of health care surrogate[9] in a Western society would be a smart legal move. Framing advance care planning around *who* will make decisions is a nice way to begin the advance care planning process with individuals who may not otherwise think that engaging in such a process is worthwhile.

Another case in which rethinking the focus of advance care planning may be helpful for a particular "target audience" involves individuals with cultural beliefs that tie the place of death to the fate of one's spirit: not an unimportant concern. As Orr explains, "individuals from some cultures place a great emphasis on where a person dies. Some believe that an individual's spirit will forever reside at the place of death, so the prospect of death in a hospital is frightening, while death at home may be quite welcome" (Orr 1996, 2005). In cases where such beliefs are operating, the focus of advance care planning can be on making explicit (e.g., through the drafting of a narrative statement) the idea that as important, indeed possibly more important than the medical treatments provided or withheld, is the goal of being at home (for instance) at the time of death. That is, an outcome-based directive could be written that emphasizes the importance of the request to die at home (or at least not in a hospital for instance). Here the advance care planning process can be driven by the concern about place of death. As such, one might request that further treatment not be provided in cases where it might serve to extend life, but require that an individual be hospitalized. In such cases the patient would have an opportunity to express a preference to forgo such medical treatments because accepting them would almost guarantee that he would not be in an acceptable location at the time of death. While the preference to not die in a hospital or any other cold, sterile health care institution tantamount to a hospital is not uncommon even amongst those who hold to the biomedical model, the reasons driving such preferences vary greatly. If a patient comes from a culture in which people do not engage in advance care planning (e.g., talking about death and dying is taboo), teasing out the preference regarding location at time of death might serve to provide a reason for engaging in such planning. Given the importance of this preference it would seem to provide a sufficient condition for broaching, in a culturally sensitive manner, the possibility of engaging in a process that would not normally even be brought up.

In such cases, the focus of advance care planning would be on making sure that treatments not preclude the possibility of an individual dying at home. As far as treatments that may have been in place for an extended period of time, an emphasis could be placed on periodic and frequent reexaminations of whether such treatments, if the patient so desired, can be continued at home. If not, then that should be made clear and alternative plans should be discussed concerning stopping such treatments that are impeding the patient's possibility of dying in an acceptable location.

In some cases, patients may be reticent to engage in advance care planning because of a lack of comfort discussing deeply personal issues, possibly any issues that stray from the "purely medical," with a health care provider. As Hudelson notes, when physicians asked patients about such things as "their personal life, migration history or war-related experiences," such questions were taken by patients to be "invasive and inappropriate in the context of a medical consultation" (Hudelson 2005, 314). Thus, in situations where the very questions foundational to productive, informative advance care planning are deemed sources of discomfort, it seems as though the advance care planning process should be avoided altogether. However, in most cases, a provider would have already begun a dialogue regarding "personal" matters with the patient before realizing that discussing such issues made the patient uncomfortable. Such an encounter may prove to be disconcerting to both patient and provider. The patient (and potentially the patient's family) might be upset, while the provider may be upset that she caused her patient distress.

By being proactive in terms of agreeing on a style of communication from the beginning of a relationship, health care providers can help to avoid some misunderstandings with patients and families. For example, providers could let patients and families know that certain questions may be seen as being of a "personal" nature, that it is standard practice to disclose information about the diagnosis and prognosis to the patient directly, and that questions and concerns about this methodology are welcome at any time. Offering this open-ended invitation for questions and concerns for even the most basic things (e.g., communication style) will help to foster a trusting relationship between patient and provider, and help to avoid conflicts that could undermine this relationship before it even begins. By being explicit about the prototypical type of conversation that occurs within the biomedical model, expectations can be set and patients and families can be encouraged to set out how they think communication between patient, family, and provider should progress. Ideally, all parties will be able to work together to determine the communication style that works best for their particular relationship. Engaging in this type of "negotiated partnership," founded on mutual respect and concern, is a good investment in terms of staving off potential conflicts, and adhering to the ideal of treating each patient as an individual. In short, the return on investing the time and energy to establish this kind of provider-patient relationship is promising and manifests a clear concern for taking seriously the practice of patient-centered care.

One of the benefits of engaging in advance care planning is that by doing so, one is able to "get things settled" or "put one's affairs in order." Value is placed on advance care planning for the opportunities it provides for patient and family to get together and discuss things that may have otherwise gone unsaid. In order for such opportunities to evolve, not only does the patient need to have information about her condition, she must also be willing to share it with friends and family. Western cultures typically applaud and encourage such openness. Indeed, there is often a great deal of effort put into creating and capitalizing on the opportunities to "make peace" before dying. Clearly, the expectations placed on these conversations are lofty. Whether it be making amends with family members or tracking down old friends to let them know that they had served as an inspiration, the importance of such opportunities should not be underemphasized. However, the high value granted to these opportunities does not hold across all cultures. Take the following case in which health care providers, who were trying to create such opportunities for a dying patient and her husband, were met with resistance and felt unappreciated and anxious about the situation:

Mrs. S is a thirty-one-year-old woman, admitted to a palliative care unit with metastatic vaginal carcinoma. . . . Both the patient and her husband are emigrants from India. She and her husband are alone in the new country (the United States), but have extensive family connections in India. Her disease has been treated locally three years prior to her admission, and has reappeared as metastases to the eye and central nervous system. The patient has advanced disease with no further anti-cancer options. She has been admitted for pain management, control of symptoms from raised intracranial pressure, and for social concerns. Her husband must continue to work, and there are no family members to help with care at home. . . . She speaks no English and her husband has limited ability to communicate in English. The patient appears to be in considerable distress but is unable to communicate the sources of her distress. . . . the patient appears to be reluctant to speak with interpreters brought in to the unit when her husband is not present. She eats very little and is restless lying in bed. . . . As her condition is rapidly declining, the staff are anxious about communication with the family. All attempts to facilitate discussion between the patient and husband were unsuccessful. Staff interpret this to mean that the patient and her husband are having great difficulty dealing with diagnosis and prognosis and are denying what is happening. Considerable concern is expressed in staff meetings that issues of closure and reconciliation with family members are not being addressed. Staff fear that the patient's denial of her condition is preventing family members who might want to speak with her the chance to do so before she dies. Repeated offers to aid in contacting distant family members are turned down. Staff are concerned about the husband who bears the burden alone, but he similarly refuses to contact his family or local friends to help him with his ordeal. (MacDonald 1998, 245–48)

Surely patient and health care provider preferences are not always coextensive. This is something that is understood in the clinical context. So, why was the staff so upset when Mrs. S and her husband refused repeated attempts to contact friends and family? Why did this difference in a preferred plan of action cause such dissonance between providers and patient? The degree of discord reflects the importance members of the health care team placed on achieving closure before death. More broadly, members of the health care team subscribed to a view in which standard practice entailed trying to address any issues that may have been left hanging, of fostering open lines of communication so as to "get things settled," of trying to make sure that death does not come before any outstanding matters are addressed. To be sure, matters concerning "closure and reconciliation" with loved ones was so much a part of what happened when someone knew she was going to die, that members of the health care team could not even fathom why Mrs. S and her husband did not jump on the chance to get in touch with their friends and family members. They assumed that the only reason one would do such a thing was because she was in denial. And, if the time came that she accepted her diagnosis and prognosis, then surely "closure and reconciliation" would be sought.

After coming to the unit and establishing a trusting relationship with the patient and her husband, a health care worker from a similar cultural background who spoke the same language was able to discern the reasoning as to why the patient and her husband did not want staff to contact family and friends. Far from being in denial about her grim prognosis, Mr. and Mrs. S were astutely aware of her condition and the potential havoc it might wreak if word got out about it back in their native village. Specifically, the health care worker learned that "in the couple's homeland it is considered a curse to die of cancer at such a young age. The patient still has three younger sisters living at home who are unmarried. Should the news of her death reach her home town, her entire family would have been considered to have been cursed, and her sisters would not have been regarded as eligible for marriage" (MacDonald 1998, 248). Thus while the benefit of having their family there for support would be great, it is outweighed by the depth and breadth of the negative consequences that would ensue if word got out about Mrs. S's condition. Given the extreme and sweeping influence such news might have on their family back in their homeland, the choice to forgo contacting friends and family to see Mrs. S before she dies and provide support to Mr. S seems quite logical. To be sure, had the couple chosen otherwise it may have seemed paradoxical and could have been construed as selfish.

Comforted by this information, the ward staff working with Mr. and Mrs. S are able to care for her without the high level of anxiety and tension that they had been feeling. No longer are they distracted by the thought of a person dying without having the opportunity to gain closure or get to say goodbye to loved ones. While it may seem as though the health care team for Mrs. S was intrusive and ought to have let the idea of contacting friends and family go after Mr. and Mrs. S made it clear that that was not what they wanted, the tenacity with which the health care team pursued this option reflects the degree of importance such actions carried and the high level of care they wanted to provide for their patient. However, the high value placed on garnering the support of loved ones, though not completely foreign to Mrs. and Mr. S, was outweighed by the importance of making sure that family back in their homeland did not suffer a tarnished reputation and retained the possibility of a future that included marriage—something very important in their culture.

Though the preferences of the patient looked vastly different than those of the health care team, the values underlying both are those that are central to the biomedical model—autonomy and beneficence. The autonomy of the patient was respected by the health care team as demonstrated by their insistence that her true desires be respected. The principle of beneficence was honored as members of the health care team went out of their way to "do good" for the patient and provide her with what they thought would be precious opportunities for closure. The patient was acting with beneficent intent, forgoing some of those precious opportunities so that her family might enjoy a future that was as open as possible. This case does well to illustrate the multifaceted nature of disclosure, caring for patients at the end of life, and the complexities that are compounded when care is provided in a pluralistic society. On a deeper level, this case highlights the importance of recognizing that some of the most fundamental issues driving advance care planning—the need to "tie up loose ends"—in some cultures might be more of an afterthought while the main goal is doing what is best for one's family as a whole. Just as easily, such issues might be seen as sources of potential harm for the family members who survive a patient's death. Contextual features of each case ought to dictate how disclosure is handled. Nonetheless, being aware of the mere possibility of such varied takes on what are deemed "fundamental values" is something that all health care providers need to have no matter the cultural background of the patient. In other words, while a health care practitioner need not know the intricacies of the beliefs and practices surrounding health care in all cultures (as this would be an unrealizable goal), she must be aware of the fact that the weight given to "core" values and how they are prioritized may vary. As such, steps must be taken to gain an understanding of where parties in the health care decision-making process are coming from, and, as much as possible, measures to accommodate various practices ought to be explored.

THINKING PRACTICALLY ABOUT
ADVANCE CARE PLANNING

Complicated, deeply personal, uncommonly broached questions with amorphous responses are the stuff of advance care planning. As such, it stands to reason that even when parties to a discussion share a similar cultural background, conflict and misunderstandings may develop. When individuals come from different cultures, with different ideas not only as to what such a conversation would look like, but whether or not it should even take place, the potential for misunderstandings and conflict is increased. Taking time to make sure that patients and providers have an idea of what the other expects—of what would be considered "protocol" to the other—is something that would be of great value. However, it is something that does take time, and the lack of time was the very issue noted earlier by a medical interpreter as posing a problem. In light of the fact that time is a scarce resource in the clinical setting, one must determine how best to use what little of it she has. Clarifying expectations is imperative. Candib notes that the onus is on the health care provider to help tease out the values and preferences of the patient. She claims that "As professionals with cultural and political power within the medical hierarchy, we must help patients and families to make explicit their values rather than expecting them to align instantly with those of the healthcare system" (Candib 2002, 225). This may lead to finding out that the patient does not want to engage in the advance care planning process at all. So too, it can allow for a plan to be developed such that patient and provider can use the time they have to the fullest. In addition, it needs to be pointed out that, even though advance care planning may sometimes begin in the clinical setting, it need not take up sole residence there. That is, the conversations at the heart of advance care planning are ones that can take place just as easily over the kitchen table as across a desk in a physician's office. In fact, the kitchen table might prove a more hospitable environment for teasing out one's values and gleaning a sense of how one would define a "good life." By starting the conversation in the clinical setting and laying the groundwork[10] for further conversations outside of the clinical setting, engaging in advance care planning may not seem like such a burden; something to detract from an already extremely limited time spent between provider and patient.

In general, whether it is an issue of how much (if any) information to disclose to the patient, how to involve family members in decision making, how to interpret body language, whether or not to ask "personal" questions, or some other issue altogether, providers should enter into relationships with patients with care. Rushing in, when the grounds on which such conversations take place are so prone to conflict, would be a foolish decision at best. Equally as bad would be to throw up one's hands and forgo attempting to engage in advance care planning, in light of the complex topography found in a diverse clinical setting. Take for instance the fact that "In certain African cultures, the traditional approach to death is not to discuss death openly or call it by that name. . . . In some cultures, the living cannot speak the names of the dead. Yet, in all African cultures, veneration, respect, and communication with the deceased are integral parts of everyday life" (Parry et al. 1995, 147). In light of this approach to death, a health care provider might deem advance care planning as something that would be too difficult to deal with and unduly time-consuming. Advance care planning is already a process that is undertaken all-too-infrequently, additional complications do not bode well in terms of increasing the frequency with which health care providers and patients undertake such an endeavor.

With additional obstacles in the way, some providers may be slow to engage in advance care planning. However, even in complex cases in which death is not discussed openly, advance care planning can be extremely valuable. Through the planning process, health care providers could still try to gauge what the patient thinks imparts value to a life, and what principles ought to guide health care treatment decisions in case of incompetence. Something as simple as making sure that loved ones are around, to making it clear that pain management ought to be a determining factor in treatment decisions, could be brought to light. For instance, ensuring that "the dying person is returned to the familiar environment of home and family to spend the last days" is of the utmost importance—especially to African American families "that have made conscious attempts to hold onto and practice the old cultural traditions" (Parry et al. 1995, 149). All of this knowledge and information could be obtained without using the word "death" or even discussing matters in terms of dying. In addition, there would be no need to use names of the deceased. Thus, even with all of the "constraints" on engaging in advance care planning, important information can still be derived that will help to draw out the treatment preferences and values of the patient. Even more, in some of the groups in which advance care planning is not normally embraced, to *not* offer such planning might be construed as an insult and an attempt to hide something from the patient. In other words, even though the patient will probably not want to draft an advance directive nor even embark on the process of advance care planning, he still would want the option to do so. He may still want to know that all of the options given to other patients are given to him as well. Simply offering the option of advance care planning is an important component in maintaining a trusting patient-provider relationship. At the end of the day, at least one shared goal of patient and provider remains—to do what is best for the patient. While engaging in advance care planning might be seen as a crucial component in obtaining this end by some, it may be seen as a likely source of conflict and tension within the patient-provider relationship. It is of the utmost importance to remember that whether or not engaging in advance care planning is seen as something that is beneficial or something that is harmful is a determination that can only be made if health care providers approach such planning and do so with care and cultural sensitivity.

NOTES

1. One of the exceptions to truth-telling in biomedicine is known as "therapeutic privilege." However, this "privilege" has come under fire as of late. See, Opinion of the Council on Ethical and Judicial Affairs, CEJA, Report 2-A-06 Withholding Information from Patients (Therapeutic Privilege).

2. As long as there is life, there is hope.

3. Clearly, there is not just one Western perspective. This is merely another case where the use of a generalization serves as an heuristic device.

4. There were both English-speaking and Japanese-speaking Japanese Americans.

5. As the case is presented, it is unclear whether or not the physician was trying to obtain this rationale over the nine-month period, or if the physician got to a point where withholding the truth from the patient, for any number of reasons, was something that would need a lot more support and justification. It is also left unclear to what extent, if at all, the physician involved the patient in deciding who would receive medical information and with whom decision-making authority would be vested. These are crucial points.

6. Specifically, Kimura quotes Ohi (1998, as quoted in Kimura) as saying that concerns were expressed regarding the "concept of a documented expression."

7. Here a living will would be appropriate, but so too would be designating a durable power attorney for health care. In such a situation, the patient could be quite specific in discussing treatment preferences with his surrogate.

8. Even if a preference is documented in a living will, it is not guaranteed, even in the biomedical model, that the wishes of the patient will be followed. This may be due to the directions in the directive being ambiguous or some other reason altogether.

9. Here, surrogate is taken to mean one who has been formally appointed to make health care decisions for the patient. This differs from the terminology in New York, for instance, where a person who is formally appointed to speak for a patient if the patient should become incompetent is called a "proxy" rather than a "surrogate."

10. Here such "groundwork" could include something like the Emanuel's Medical Directive or The Five Wishes from Aging With Dignity.

Chapter Five

Realizing the Goal of Cultural Sensitivity in the Clinical Setting— Where the Rubber Hits the Road

If we are to achieve a richer culture, rich in contrasting values, we must recognize the whole gamut of human potentialities, and so weave a less arbitrary social fabric, one in which each diverse gift will find a fitting place.

—Margaret Mead

I want all the cultures of all lands to be blown about my house as freely as possible. But I refuse to be blown off my feet by any.

—Mahatma Gandhi

When I began working on this book, a research assistant of mine shared with me a picture of what she thought the provision of health care ought to look like. At the core was the idea that everyone be treated as a unique individual. Not a new idea, nor a controversial supposition, but one that is too often forgotten in the fast-paced clinical setting where time is one of the scarcest resources of all. One of the most striking things about the picture she described was how much sense it made. How simple it appeared, and yet, seeing it in practice seemed too often an anomaly. She explained how she, a middle class, Caucasian, college-educated female wanted health care providers to approach her the same way that they would approach, for instance, an elderly, Spanish-speaking, Cuban man. Primarily, she was concerned that the way a health care provider approached a patient not be dictated by whether or not English was a first or second language, or by whether one has been in the United States (for instance) for a year or for his whole life. Rather, health care providers need to stop assuming that people come to health encounters from a position of sameness and begin to approach everyone with a spirit of inquiry. Awareness of one's own lens through which the world is viewed, coupled with the recognition of the plurality of other world views, will hopefully lead to the practice of health care in which patient and provider meet with an expectation of mutual discovery and individualized care. Culturally sensitive health care is not something that should be engaged in only when patient and provider are from different cultures. Instead, it should be a standard of care—a threshold below which a good provider ought not fall. In short, "The main rule is that there is no rule. Treat each person as an individual. We must *ask* how we may help and we must *listen* to the response. Our mere presence as a person who cares, will be a significant starting point" (Taylor et al. 1999, 13 of 54).

IF YOU GIVE A MAN A FISH . . .

The call for increased cultural sensitivity amongst health care providers must be coupled with a plan of action. It would be unfulfilling at least and possibly unfair to demonstrate the immense importance of increasing cultural sensitivity and not, at the same time, offer guidance on how to achieve such a goal. To be sure, there is no one algorithm, no single method that would furnish health care providers with all the tools necessary for successful cross-cultural interactions. However, there are several tools aimed at increasing cultural sensitivity that are available. It is in the spirit of respecting each person as an individual and, hopefully, decreasing the incidence of conflict born out of cross-cultural misunderstandings that I have gathered these tools. While these tools have already been developed, there is still much value to be gained in commenting on and compiling them in one place for quick reference. In addition, compiling these various approaches to cross-cultural communication provides one with an opportunity to pick and choose which approach (or combination thereof) would best fit one's situation. Taking into account things like patient demographics and past conflicts born out of cultural differences will help providers tailor an approach for their particular practice. Whether one is practicing in a rural community hospital, a large, urban research institution, with a primarily geriatric or solely pediatric population, or in some other setting altogether, having so many options available will facilitate a more informed decision concerning how best to approach increasing the level of cultural sensitivity in the provision of health care. Even more, I have tried to include those guidelines that can be woven with ease into the fabric of medical practice. As Searight et al. note,

> Although cultural proficiency guidelines exist, few resources are available to family physicians regarding ways to apply these guidelines to direct patient care. Many physicians are unfamiliar with common cultural variations regard-

ing physician-patient communication, medical decision making, and attitudes about formal documents such as code status guidelines and advance directives. End-of-life discussions are particularly challenging because of their emotional and interpersonal intensity. (Searight et al. 2005, 515)

The following sections are offered in hopes of answering this call to provide tools that are easy to operationalize from the systems level to the bedside.

THE PLAN

While efforts have been put forth to prepare health care providers for practice in a pluralistic clinical setting, until fairly recently such efforts have been more akin to providing them with something like a card catalogue of various cultures and their respective beliefs and practices regarding health care. First, such a "resource" would be incomplete at best and serve to foster a false sense of comfort for health care providers operating in a culturally diverse clinical setting. To think that one could learn about (to say nothing of truly understanding) all of the details surrounding health care for all of the different cultures one may encounter in the clinical setting would be either hubristic or delusional. Either way, it would not be possible. Rather than encourage such a futile endeavor, what I aim to do in this chapter is to provide various resources on which providers can draw and develop a way to approach their patients in a culturally sensitive manner, setting the foundation for strong patient–health care provider relationships.

One of the interesting things to note about the various tools for facilitating a greater level of culturally sensitive care is that they are all quite compatible with being used in a setting in which autonomy is the most highly prized value. This becomes apparent as soon as one realizes that in order to operate within a pluralistic clinical setting, one needs to adopt a broader, more robust conception of autonomy. If we do value autonomy—and it seems clear that we do—then such a reconceptualization must occur. More broadly, in a world in which relationships are constantly being forged and we are becoming increasingly more interconnected, adopting a more robust conception of autonomy secures for one a greater likelihood of success in terms of navigating complex clinical waters. In the face of the plurality of views on how to discuss, treat, and live and die with illness, it should be clear that the goals of health care providers must not, indeed cannot, conform to some ideal created by the biomedical model. Instead, we must cultivate ways of delivering health care that respect the current norms, and at the same time, allow room for individuals from other cultures to obtain healthcare in a way that accords with their deeply held cultural practices and beliefs.

In the first section of this chapter I offer several tools that have been developed to help direct practitioners on how to engage in culturally sensitive communication in general. Tools include the "Four Fundamental Principles for Better Communication" from Oncotalk, "Guidelines for Making End-of-Life Care More Culturally Sensitive" from Werth et al., Leininger's Short Culturologic Assessment in Wright et al., Spector's considerations for approaching patients in a culturally sensitive manner, the LEARN model from Berlin and Fowkes, and the Eight Questions from Kleinman et al. While patient participation in health care decision making is a mainstay in these tools, it is something that is offered to patients as opposed to forced on them. Offering participation in treatment decisions can be taken as something similar to Freedman's "offering truth" model of delivering information to a patient.[1] In Freedman's model, the truth about the diagnosis and prognosis is not thrust on the patient regardless of whether or not the patient wanted such information. Rather, "a patient will be offered the opportunity to learn the truth, at whatever level of detail that patient desires. The most important step in these attempts to "offer truth" is to ask questions of the patient and then listen closely to the patient's responses" (Freedman, 113, in Steinbock et al. 2008). In culturally sensitive health care decision making, patient participation is not mandatory. It is seen as a "right" rather than a "duty" (Freedman in Steinbock et al. 2008).

Next, I will focus on tools that will be useful specifically for engaging in culturally sensitive advance care planning. Tools here include the Giger-Davidhizar Transcultural Model, Taylor and Cameron's Five Steps in an Idealized Process of Advance Care Planning, Pearls/Ideas to Facilitate Conversations about Goals of Care from Oncotalk, and a Checklist for the Planning of End-Of-Life Decisions in Patients with a Terminal Disease from Voltz et al. Recognition of the fact that advance care planning is not necessarily a benign process that individuals may take or leave is a necessary first step in developing a way to approach such planning in a culturally sensitive manner. Awareness of this fact may make some health care providers even more reluctant to broach the issue of advance care planning. Given that advance care planning is already a topic on which health care providers may be reticent to initiate a dialogue with patients, additional reasons for them not to start such conversations serve to stand in the way of what could be very important, informative discussions. However, the potential dangers imbedded in issues common to advance care planning are intertwined with the potential for fruitful conversations and strengthened provider-patient relationships. The best course for determining how to derive these benefits of the advance care planning process and at the same time decrease the likelihood of incurring the burdens is to approach such discussions in a culturally sensitive manner. In an effort to chart such a course, I will examine efforts to develop culturally sensitive educational materials that providers can use to help communicate with patients in a pluralistic setting, and offer some ideas as to how to focus future efforts in this area.

It is important to note that while increasing the level of cultural sensitivity of providers is extremely important, it is not the only component in increasing the overall level of cultural sensitivity in an organization. With this goal in mind—increasing the overall level of cultural sensitivity—the next section on how to develop and identify a culturally sensitive organization is offered. Finally, in an effort to determine how effective various efforts to increase cultural sensitivity at all levels of a health care institution have been, some points for consideration during assessment are offered. Ultimately, this section identifies areas in which increasing the level of culturally sensitive care is important, provides tools to use in achieving this goal, and ways to measure how successful various measures have been.

MODELS FOR FACILITATING
CULTURALLY SENSITIVE COMMUNICATION

A useful first step in beginning to increase the level of cultural sensitivity in a health care institution is to assess the needs of the particular organization at issue. This will allow a more focused effort and, hopefully, avoid wasting time that is already very limited. Though it may seem self-evident, one part of such an assessment needs to be obtaining and keeping data on the cultural groups served by the institution. Such data should be available within the hospital. In addition, state-level data on things such as prevalence and incidence of certain diseases within a population[2] and composition of various populations,[3] are available on the internet. Not only should the needs of an institution be assessed based on the demographic picture obtained, but also, at the same time, by the specific concerns and interests voiced by the populations served by the institution. That is, one should not merely obtain information on, for instance, how much of the patient population served is made up of African Americans, Native Americans, etc. While such data is useful in combination with other information, by itself it does not provide too much insight into how to increase the level of cultural sensitivity throughout the organization. After obtaining an overview of the patient population served, one needs to then delve into the needs and interests of such populations.

An important component of any plan aimed at increasing the level of cultural sensitivity in an institution is to invite participation from the community. To begin with, community members can provide valuable, firsthand insight into the issues they deem pressing in health care. Not only can information on what issues are important be obtained, but so too, valuable insight into how such issues are understood and faced within the community can also be derived. Including community members at the outset in developing methods of increasing cultural sensitivity reveals a good faith effort to establish a partnership with the community and gives members of the community "buy in" to any methods that are developed, helping to create a sense of ownership of any policies or procedures that may evolve. The data regarding the cultural diversity of the patient population served by a particular health care institution is also useful in directing resources and focusing attention at various levels of the institution. For instance, in a hospital where a large portion of the patient population is Hispanic, more resources could be directed toward programs focusing on increasing understanding and awareness of some of the beliefs and practices of that culture.

Several tools have been developed to help facilitate culturally sensitive communication at the patient-provider level (table 5.1). Foundational to any attempt to foster culturally sensitive communication is becoming a good communicator in general. One approach for more effective communication has been developed by Oncotalk.[4] Though this program was developed specifically to help medical oncologists communicate with their patients, its message is generalizable to a broad range of health care providers. Specifically, I will focus on one of the principles noted in the "Four Fundamental Principles for Better Communication," the "Ask-Tell-Ask" principle. Briefly, this principle instructs providers on how to engage their patients in a dialogue and facilitate the sharing of information between parties. To begin, the provider is to "*ASK* the patient to describe her current understanding of the issue" (Fryer-Edwards et al. 2002, Module 1). Next, the provider is to "*TELL* the patient in straightforward language what [the provider] needs to communicate—the bad news, or treatment options, or other information" (Fryer-Edwards et al. 2002, Module 1). Finally, the provider is to "*ASK* the patient if she understood what [the provider] just said" (Fryer-Edwards et al. 2002, Module 1). In addition, this model goes further in guiding providers in how to deal with situations in which they get "stuck" or if the conversation begins to go astray. It also helps providers "respond to emotion" and "assess the patient's coping style" (Fryer-Edwards et al. 2002, Module 1). Of note with this model is its focus on shared communication and a partnership between patient and provider aimed at developing a common understanding of the situation, coupled with a mutual effort to establish a treatment plan. Right away, a provider is given some indication of her patient's comfort level. If the patient seems quite shy and uneasy when "*ASKED*" to offer his understanding of the situation, the provider can take a more active role in asking questions, rather than expect the patient to offer up a long, involved narrative. While the provider must still afford the pa-

Table 5.1:   General Cultural Sensitivity Tools

Tool Name	Key Components of Tool	Benefits of Tool	Settings in which Tool Is Most Useful
"Four Fundamental Principles for Better Communication" from Oncotalk (Module 1) (Fryer-Edwards et al. 2002)	"Ask-Tell-Ask" principle - "*ASK* the patient to describe her current understanding of the issue" - "*TELL* the patient in straightforward language what [the provider] needs to communicate- the bad news, or treatment options, or other information" - "*ASK* the patient if she understood what [the provider] just said"	- focus on shared communication and a partnership between patient and provider - goal of developing a common understanding of the situation - helps providers "respond to emotion" - helps providers "assess the patient's coping style"	- guidance is general enough to be used across various settings (e.g., outpatient and acute care settings; general practitioners and subspecialists)
"Guidelines for Making End-of-Life Care More Culturally Sensitive" from Werth et al. (compilation) (Werth et al. 2002)	- Determine the locus of decision making - Assess the degree of fatalism or activism within the patient and family - Assess how hope is maintained within the family and negotiated with health care providers - Solicit information from all possible sources within the community	- directs providers to take a more robust view of the patient, allowing patients to be viewed within a context, within a narrative (e.g., providers are instructed to "consider sociopolitical and historical factors that influence beliefs about illness, health care, and death, such as poverty, refugee status, past discrimination, and issues related to access to health care" - highlights very particular issues and areas on which to focus when practicing in a diverse clinical context	- wonderful to use with new patients in order to establish a baseline and gain important information about how to proceed with caring for the "patient as a person" - prompts are general enough to be used not only across specialties, but across disciplines (e.g., physians, nurses, clinical social workers, etc.)

Table 5.1: General Cultural Sensitivity Tools (continued)

Tool Name	Key Components of Tool	Benefits of Tool	Settings in which Tool Is Most Useful
Wright et al., on Leininger's Short Culturologic Assessment (Wright et al. 1997)	- "recording observations" from interactions with patients, emphasis is also placed on letting the patient tell her story and learning directly from the patient about the patient	- picks up on the value of simply observing the patient - highlights importance of documenting the meanings of what has been seen/heard/said according to the patient - providers need to be conscious of what patients and families are saying about the context from which they come	- very good to use with patients that are seen on a continuous basis, to watch for consistency (or lack thereof) of preferences
Spector's considerations for approaching patients in a culturally sensitive manner (Spector 2003)	- establish how patient prefers to be addressed - careful of what you may be saying with body language - speak directly to the patient - determine the reading comprehension level of the patient before providing written materials	- provides clear, specific instruction on fundamental issues, including basics such as where in the room the patient would feel most comfortable being seated	- wonderful for use with new patients
Berlin and Fowkes, LEARN Model (Berlin and Fowkes 1983)	- Listen, Explain, Acknowledge, Recommend, Negotiate	-used as a "supplement" to the medical interview -useful in determining the patient's understanding of his illness -good tool for allowing the patient to be an active participant in developing his own medical treatment plan	-good to use with a new patient or a patient that has been seen before in order to establish where patient is at in terms of his understanding of his medical situation

Table 5.1:   General Cultural Sensitivity Tools (continued)

Tool Name	Key Components of Tool	Benefits of Tool	Settings in which Tool Is Most Useful
Kleinman's "Eight Questions" (Kleinman et al. 1978)	- eight questions that help provider gain insight into patient's understanding of the sickness (e.g., what caused it, how it "works," etc.) - questions also pinpoint specific fears of the patient and sets out prompts for providers to identify and explore the goals of treatment	- Introduces idea of "explanatory model of illness" - points out the vast differences in how individuals may approach illness and reminds providers that patients are often coming to the encounter with different understandings of sickness	- useful in a wide variety of settings including (but not limited to) inpatient and outpatient hospital settings, clinic visits, and routine office visits

tient with opportunities to take a more active role in the dialogue, it is up to the patient to determine whether or not to seize such opportunities. Ultimately, the onus is on the provider to gain insight into the patient's understanding of the situation. Where differences in understanding exist, both patient and provider need to work to convey their respective views. Here, being open to different ways of understanding illness and how to cope with it is paramount. Both patient and provider need to work together to develop a treatment plan that is neither imposed by the provider on the patient, nor demanded inflexibly by the patient, but rather constructed by both parties through a process of mutual cooperation and shared understanding. Overall, this principle makes explicit the need for all parties in the decision-making process to try and understand the various perspectives being brought to the table.

Werth et al. put together a valuable compilation of suggestions for increasing cultural sensitivity in end-of-life care from several sources. Some of the suggestion include:

- Assess the language that the patient/family use in discussing the illness and disease, including the extent of openness with regard to the diagnosis, prognosis, and death.
- Determine the locus of decision making. Is it the individual patient, the family, or another social unit?
- Solicit the patient's and family's views about the appropriate location and timing of death, including the preferred role of family members and health care providers.

- Assess the degree of fatalism or activism within the patient and family. Is there acceptance regarding future events or a desire to control aspects of these events?
- Assess religious beliefs of the patient and family, focusing on the meaning of death, the existence of an afterlife, and belief in miracles. Also, establish beliefs about the body after death (e.g., who owns the body and how is it to be treated?).
- Assess how hope is maintained within the family and negotiated with health care providers. What are the cultural meanings associated with maintaining hope?
- Consider sociopolitical and historical factors that influence beliefs about illness, health care, and death, such as poverty, refugee status, past discrimination, and issues related to access to health care (Werth et al. 2002, 214).[5]

This list provides significant guidance in helping to determine the cultural perspective a patient is coming from when trying to decide what her medical treatment should look like at the end of life. One of the benefits of these suggestions is that they highlight very particular issues and areas on which to focus when practicing in a diverse clinical context. Simply by mentioning various issues (e.g., does the family take a fatalistic attitude toward future events), it raises the awareness of the health care provider, and, in many cases, may place on her radar things that would have otherwise been overlooked. At the same time, the prompts are general enough to be used not only across specialties, but across disciplines. Issues touched on in Werth's list are important to everyone charged with caring for the patient, from the physician, to the social worker, to the nutritionist. While some of these suggestions will be repeated in other models that are included in this chapter, such repetition is not an oversight. Rather, it should serve to underscore the importance of the suggestions, in that multiple authors have noted the need to include them in methods focused on approaching health care in a culturally sensitive manner.

In their work on increasing culturally sensitivity in health care, Wright et al. bring in and promote Leininger's Short Culturologic Assessment, in which there is a "framework for assessment versus a checklist of questions" (Wright et al. 1997, 72).[6] While Wright et al. direct their article to critical care nurses, the guidance they provide is applicable to a wide range of health care providers working in a multicultural setting. Wright et al. go through several components of Leininger's assessment framework. They highlight the importance of seemingly simple practices—from simple observation of how patients behave to listening carefully to what patients have to say—practices that health care providers can easily overlook. In addition to "recording observations" from interactions with patients, emphasis is also placed on letting the patient tell her story and learning directly from the patient about the patient (Wright et al. 1997, 72). Even more than simply observing patients as acting in a particular way at a particular time, Wright et al. bring out the idea, from the Leininger model, that providers should focus on "Identifying and documenting *recurrent* client patterns and stories with client meanings of what has been seen, heard and experienced" (Wright et al. 1997, 72, emphasis added). Learning about the patient does not necessarily occur solely by means of the patient telling the provider about himself directly. Instead, as the Leininger model points out, such knowledge can be obtained through observation of how a patient acts or from gleaning insight from general stories that a patient tells. A nice feature of this approach is the active role the health care provider needs to assume in approaching care for her patient, as opposed to simply treating a disease. It is the provider who needs to be vigilant for anything that might help her to better understand her patients. Such vigilance can pay off exponentially in terms of better communication with patients. In addition, this approach helps to remind providers to be aware of patient preferences and values and to note whether or not they change over time. If such changes occur, this can prompt further investigation as to why such changes have occurred. Also beneficial, is the call for providers to be sensitive to indicators beyond clinical signs and symptoms. On this approach, providers need to be conscious of what patients and families are saying about the context from which they come, their history, their place in the present, and where they see themselves in the future.

Another nice tool aimed at "enhancing communication" in a pluralistic clinical setting is put forth by Spector (Spector 2003, 325). Spector offers several points to consider in approaching patients in a culturally sensitive manner. Ideally, by keeping such points in mind the relationship between patient and provider will run smoothly and a greater level of understanding, for both parties, can be achieved (Spector 2003, 325):

- Determine the level of fluency in English and arrange for a competent interpreter, when needed.
- Ask how the patient prefers to be addressed.
- Allow the patient to choose seating for comfortable personal space and eye contact. If the patient prefers to *not* establish eye contact, do not become upset. In many cultures it is considered polite to avoid eye contact.
- Avoid body language and gestures that may be offensive or misunderstood.
- Speak directly and quietly to the patient, whether an interpreter is present or not.

- Choose a speech rate and style that promotes understanding and demonstrates respect for the patient.
- Avoid slang, technical jargon, and complex sentences.
- Use open-ended questions or questions phrased in several ways to obtain information.
- Determine the patient's reading ability before using written materials in the teaching process.
- Provide reading material that is easily read in the patient's native language. Do not use cartoons and cartoon characters for illustrations.

Here, Spector provides guidance at both a specific and at a quite general level. The specific points of guidance are wonderful insofar as they allow health care providers to rule certain practices in (or out) right away in their quest to increase their level of cultural sensitivity. Benefits of her more general guidance include the ability to employ these guidelines and capitalize on them in a variety of different settings. That is, one can use them in an inpatient or outpatient setting, with general medicine or with subspecialties, in a rural or urban health care institution, etc. For instance, Spector gives providers wonderful guidance by simply reminding providers to ask patients how they would like to be addressed. If a provider addresses a patient in a way that the patient feels is too informal, it might be construed as disrespectful and the patient may not even want to continue on in a relationship with a provider whom he feels does not treat him with respect. Similarly, if the provider addresses a patient in a manner that the patient feels is overly formal, the patient may feel uncomfortable and not want to engage in a dialogue with the provider and share personal details—details necessary for offering proper health care to a patient. Overall, Spector makes it clear that the patient is the best resource for direction on how to treat the patient. Providers would do well to let the patient establish things like the pace of the conversation, the level of formality (i.e., in terms of how to be addressed), all the way to the amount of space to be maintained between patient and provider during discussions. Looking to the patient for guidance on such issues can help make the patient more comfortable and allow for a better health care experience overall for both patient and provider.

Another useful tool for approaching a patient in a culturally sensitive way in order to elicit his understanding of the situation and gather valuable information on how to care for him is the LEARN model developed by Berlin and Fowkes. LEARN stands for:

- *Listen* with sympathy and understanding to the patient's perception of the problem
- *Explain* your perceptions of the problem

- *Acknowledge* and discuss the differences and similarities
- *Recommend* treatment
- *Negotiate* agreement (Berlin and Fowkes 1983, 934)

Berlin and Fowkes maintain that instead of a replacement for "the normal structure of the medical interview," the LEARN model is more of a "supplement" to the medical interview focused on determining the "patient's theoretical explanation of the reasons for the problem" (Berlin and Fowkes 1983, 935). Emphasizing the importance not only of appreciating the patient's perception of the illness and the course thereof, but also of making clear the provider's understanding of the illness, sets the stage for a relationship based on clear lines of communication and mutual understanding. Such a foundation is ideal for engaging in developing, recommending, and negotiating treatment plans. When both patient and provider are active participants in developing a treatment plan, both have a stake in the final product and the process is much more balanced than it would be if parties were coming to the table with vast disparities in their level of understanding of the situation. As such, a sense of ownership on the part of provider *and* patient is established. The treatment plan is no longer something that is thrust on a patient, but rather, something which the patient had an integral part in developing. With a product that is "an amalgamation resulting from a unique partnership in decision making between provider and patient," patients will be better positioned to follow the plans and incorporate them into their lives (Berlin and Fowkes 1983, 935). Overall, the LEARN model furnishes providers with prompts that when incorporated into patient-provider relationship, facilitate an environment of mutual discovery, understanding, and respect between patient and provider.

One of the classic tools to help providers practice culturally sensitive care and gain insight into how the patient understands his illness is a set of eight questions put forth by Kleinman et al. Compiling answers to these questions allows the provider to construct the "patient's explanatory model" of illness. Overall, "the patient model gives the physician knowledge of the beliefs the patient holds about his illness, the personal and social meaning he attaches to his disorder, his expectations about what will happen to him and what the doctor will do, and his own therapeutic goals" (Kleinman et al. 1978, 256). By constructing and exploring the patient's explanatory model, the health care provider is better able to determine which parts of her own model and the patient's model do not align and work to reconcile such differences (e.g., through additional patient education) (Kleinman et al. 1978). Kleinman et al. offer the following eight questions in an effort to understand a patient and elucidate how she perceives the situation, what values are driving her preferences, and what it is she hopes to achieve through her treatment choices[7]:

1. What do you think has caused your problem?
2. Why do you think it started when it did?
3. What do you think your sickness does to you? How does it work?
4. How severe is your sickness? Will it have a short or long course?
5. What kind of treatment do you think you should receive?
6. What are the most important results you hope to receive from this treatment?
7. What are the chief problems your sickness has caused for you?
8. What do you fear most about your sickness? (Kleinman et al. 1978, 256)

The first five questions help a provider demonstrate to a patient that the patient's ideas are "of genuine interest and importance for clinical management," while questions six through eight help to "Elicit the patient's therapeutic goals and the psychosocial and cultural meaning of his illness (Kleinman et al. 1978, 256). These questions help to establish a solid foundation composed of a shared understanding between patient and provider. Another benefit of these questions is that they are general enough to be used in a variety of settings (e.g., in a hospital, a routine office visit, etc.), but they are not so general that they lack the power to derive useful information from patients. Not only do these questions provide basic information around notions of what the patient believes caused the sickness and what the patient thinks would be good treatment options (all very important issues) they also strike at a fundamental motivating factor in why a patient chooses as he does—fear. By identifying what it is that the patient fears most, the provider can focus on alleviating that fear and dispelling any misunderstandings that surround the patient's fears. This will help to decrease the level of patient anxiety and foster a more relaxed atmosphere in which to concentrate on caring for the patient and in which the patient can focus on matters other than unfounded fears. Clearly, while some fears may in fact be unfounded, other fears may not. If in fact there are grounds for a patient to have a particular fear, it is useful simply to get this fear out into the open and alert the provider to the primacy it has been granted by the patient. In addition to the therapeutic value of "being heard," making clear what is feared most about the sickness can help patient and provider work together to develop a treatment plan in which efforts to address certain fears are given priority. Overall these eight questions equip providers in a variety of settings with the tools necessary to begin a discussion with patients that has as its goal a mutually agreeable treatment plan based on understanding and appreciation of the views of all parties involved in the decision-making process.

While adaptability is a benefit of any tool, the same qualities (namely, generality) that allow for such adaptability can also prove to be a bit of a drawback. Most notably, health care providers, in consulting such models, are looking for guidance on how to practice in a pluralistic setting. If the models are very general, they may not be as helpful as they could be in directing patient care. What is important to note about the models discussed in this section is that not any one of the models taken in isolation is exhaustive. By taking the most applicable parts of each model and combining them to work best for one's circumstances, health care providers can tailor their own guides. Determining which practices are most appropriate involves reflecting on the patient populations being served, making sure to engage in continuing education to achieve and maintain culturally sensitive practices, and becoming aware of the various resources[8] (both within the health care institution and in the broader community) available to help in caring for patients in a multicultural context. The importance of consulting broadly and utilizing a variety of resources cannot be overemphasized. Ultimately, any amalgamation of parts of these tools should aim for the goal of fewer conflicts and greater satisfaction on the part of both patients and providers. One area where the potential for conflicts is quite high is advance care planning. As such, developing tools that are aimed specifically at helping facilitate the advance care planning process, particularly in a pluralistic clinical context, is extremely useful.

CS MODELS FOR ADVANCE CARE PLANNING

Advance directives are founded on an edifice composed of Western values, focused primarily on patient autonomy.[9] As a result, advance care planning and advance directives are not universally recognized nor are they always understood. Frequently, parties engaging in the process of advance care planning are starting at deeply varied positions of understanding. Taking time to explain the process and making the patient comfortable are crucial components of successful advance care planning. One way of making the patient feel more comfortable is to work on becoming a good listener, allowing the patient to tell his story, to elucidate his values and make his preferences known. In short, allow ample opportunities, which the patient may or may not want to take advantage of, for the patient to be heard. Allowing a patient to tell his story, if he so chooses, is but a first step in fostering an environment conducive to successful advance care planning.

Refraining from jumping to judgment is another important component in facilitating an open and honest discussion in which to explore deeply personal issues so critical in successful advance care planning. Take for example a case in which a patient, in discussing her experiences with death and dying, reveals a belief system[10] that includes spirits and visions:

A few years ago I had a young cousin who was living in New York and who died of AIDS. This was before the medication AZT was on the market, so the course of the disease was relatively short from the time of diagnosis to the time of demise. The week before he died, his mother began to have a series of dreams in which I placed an urgent call to her to come to New York because her son was dying. She later saw me, in the vision, accompanying the casket back to our home town in Virginia. This young man was not known to have any illness. A week later, these same events happened almost exactly as in his mother's dreams, which she revealed to me a couple of weeks after his death. (Parry and Ryan 1995, 153)

Showing a willingness to listen to and learn about things like visions and spirits, things that are not often welcomed from a scientific, biomedical perspective, will allow the patient to feel more comfortable with the provider and develop a trusting relationship. Non-judgmental engagement and careful listening might allow for information to be shared and plans to be made based on information that might never have been relayed had the patient and family not trusted the health care provider enough to open up. The culturally sensitive provider will work to understand and appreciate information given to her. The anecdote above stands as a perfect opportunity to gain insight into the patient's thoughts on what was good and/or bad about the circumstances under which her cousin died, and reflect on how these judgments might influence her own preferences for care at the end of life. Approaching patients with a spirit of inquiry and working with them to gain an understanding of their situation, even when such understanding is obtained through what may be seen as unconventional means (e.g., discussing visions and talking about ancestral spirits), will allow for the greatest opportunity to develop a robust advance care plan.

Specific tools have been developed to help providers engage in culturally sensitive advance care planning (table 5.1). The Giger-Davidhizar Transcultural Model is a sort of hybrid—a tool that is as good at improving communication between patient and provider in general as it is for setting the groundwork for a culturally sensitive, informed conversation on advance care planning. As a setup to their model, Giger et al. (2006) note how important it is that when approaching a patient, the health care provider must leave behind "pre-conceived ideas" about the patient's culture. In addition, two crucial questions for a provider to keep in mind when trying to gain an understanding of how the patient understands the situation are, "What is your greatest concern?" and "How can I be of help?" (Giger et al. 2006, 7). These two questions make it possible so that "care can begin with what the patient feels is the greatest priority" (Giger et al. 2006, 7).

Table 5.2: Tools for Culturally Sensitive Advance Care Planning

Tool Name	Key Components of Tool	Benefits of Tool	Settings in which Tool Is Most Useful
Giger-Davidhizar Transcultural Model (Giger et al. 2006 and Giger and Davidhizar 2002)	- highlights two basic questions that can help foster a more productive, smoother advance care planning process: (1) "What is your greatest concern?" and (2) "How can I be of help?" - provides a useful framework around which patient assessment can be conducted	- helps determine important, but often overlooked "environmental" details of the patient-provider interaction (e.g., amount of space to maintain between patient and provider, whether the patient's manner is "stoic" or "expressive") - provides specific, helpful guiding questions	- useful for guidance in general patient-provider communication - very useful in engaging in the advance care planning process (e.g., helps determine with whom decision-making authority rests)
Taylor and Cameron: list of five steps in an idealized process of advance care planning (Taylor and Cameron 2002)	(i) Raising the topic and giving information, (ii) Facilitating a structured discussion, (iii) Completing a statement and recording it, (iv) Periodically reviewing and updating the directives, and (v) Bringing prior wishes to bear on actual decisions	- provides guidance in terms of order in which to embark on the advance care planning process - prompts providers to revisit directives and not allow them to become dated and a poor representation of patient preferences	- good for broaching advance care planning process with patients—but only if done so in a culturally sensitive manner
Oncotalk: Pearls/Ideas to Facilitate Conversations about Goals of Care (Module 4) (Fryer-Edwards et al. 2002)	- offers specific "phrases that might be helpful" for engaging in the advance care planning process	- provides crucial reminder for providers to establish a clear understanding of the patient's goals - makes explicit the fact that engaging in advance care planning is an opportunity not an obligation for patients	- can help providers in general (as establishing the patient's goals is always important)

Table 5.2: Tools for Culturally Sensitive Advance Care Planning (continued)

Tool Name	Key Components of Tool	Benefits of Tool	Settings in which Tool Is Most Useful
		- points out that providers need to thank patients and families for engaging in advance care planning and sharing intimate details surrounding treatment preferences at the end of life	- quite valuable in engaging in the advance care planning process and elucidating helpful details in terms of what a good/bad death would look like for a paitent - very useful in determining what is driving patient preferences, thus allowing providers to understand and appreciate why a patient chooses as he does
Voltz et al., in their Checklist for Planning of End-of-Life Decisions in Patients with a Terminal Disease (Volts et al. 1998)	- offers providers open-ended questions (good for entering into the advance care planning process), leaving room for patients to explain their preferences and values to health care providers	- prompts health care providers to ask some very basic, very important questions - drawn from research done in the United States, Germany, and Japan	- useful in advance care planning, specifically in determining fundamental issues (e.g., whether the patient would prefer to receive care at home or in hospital)

In general, the Giger-Davidhizar Transcultural Model "includes six cultural phenomena: communication, time, space, social organization, environmental control, and biological variations. These provide a framework for patient assessment and from which culturally sensitive care can be designed" (Giger et al. 2002, 185). Not only does this model delineate useful cultural phenomena under which to organize data pertinent to assessing a patient's cultural beliefs, but it also provides health care practitioners with various questions to prompt patients and families for the information necessary to add the flesh to the bones of the framework. (Giger et al. 2006). Questions are grouped by topic, and then subsumed under each of the six categories.[11] For example, one topic Giger and Davidhizar list is end-of-life decision making. Under the "communication" category, questions relating to the end of life include (but are not limited to), "Who is the decision maker in the family?" "Does the individual have a stoic or expressive manner?" and "Are questions asked freely or only after trust is developed?" (Giger et al. 2006, 8). The answers to these questions will help providers ascertain how best to engage the patient in a dialogue, thus helping to establish a rapport with patients. And, by communicating in the manner most amendable to the patient (as determined through asking the "communication" questions), health care providers can maximize the amount of information relayed by the patient and, at the same time, increase the amount of information received and understood by the patient.

Questions concerning how much (if at all) family closeness is valued are asked under the category "space," while issues of whether "the individual [is] past, present, or future-oriented?" are considered under the category "time" (Giger et al. 2006, 8). Answers to questions under the "space" and "time" categories can provide valuable insight into who should be included in the advance care planning process and whether or not such a future-directed process makes sense in the worldview of certain individuals. Under the "environmental control" category, health care providers try and determine where the locus of control resides. That is, is there an internal locus of control wherein the individual has a great deal of "power to affect change," or is the locus of control external in which case "luck . . . and chance have a great deal to do with how things turn out" (Giger et al. 2006, 8)? In terms of "social organization," questions focus on issues such as whether individuals "believe in a supreme being," the religious beliefs of the individual, and how the individual identifies his "assigned role" in his family (i.e., does he identify himself as a son, husband, etc. . . .)" (Giger et al. 2006, 8). Finally, questions under the "biological variations" category center on determining the "health status of the individual," asking whether "pain is expressed freely or only when asked," and gauging what level of pain, if any, the individual believes "should be tolerated" (Giger et al. 2006, 8).

One of the most valuable aspects of this model is that in addition to providing guiding questions, Giger and Davidhizar offer categories under which to organize the information collected. With the immense amount of data that can be derived from employing the Giger-Davidhizar model, having some way to organize it is quite important. Organizational categories will help to ensure that data can be accessed easily and quickly. The facility with which one is able to access data is important in the clinical setting where time is already very limited. Taking the time to understand the patient's perspective serves as evidence that the provider aims to care for the patient in a way that respects the patient's beliefs and values. Hopefully patients and families take advantage of proactive health care providers and work to make their values and preferences as clear as possible. Ultimately, with all parties working to engage in a mutually respectful, culturally sensitive health care encounter, the chance for conflict born out of cultural misunderstandings will be minimized.

While the Giger-Davidhizar model is a useful tool for increasing cultural sensitivity in general communication, the questions it provides and the categories it demarcates are also quite valuable for approaching issues in advance care planning. For instance, simply by determining who the decision maker is in the family, health care providers can (with the patient's permission) invite this person to be a part of advance care planning discussions and gain clarity in general regarding which parties are to be part of the advance care planning process. In addition, being open to inviting loved ones into the advance care planning process indicates to loved ones that providers are amenable to including them in the conversation and, in fact, see them as important sources of information in developing an end-of-life treatment plan. Ultimately, this tool, along with all of the others mentioned thus far, is only as good as the provider using it. The more aware the provider is of the differences that may exist and of the manner in which these sensitive questions ought to be broached, the greater success she will have in obtaining valuable insight that can serve to make the health care encounter smoother and allow the patient and provider to feel as though they have been a part of a mutually respectful relationship.

In addition to tools that can be used for more general conversations as well as conversations that focus on advance care planning, tools targeted specifically for use in advance care planning have also been put forward. Taylor and Cameron describe a list of five steps in an idealized process of advance care planning:

(i)   Raising the topic and giving information,
(ii) Facilitating a structured discussion,
(iii) Completing a statement and recording it,
(iv) Periodically reviewing and updating the directives, and
(v)   Bringing prior wishes to bear on actual decisions. (Taylor et al. 2002, 476)

This model provides a nice guide in terms of the order in which to proceed when engaging in advance care planning. It does well not only to remind practitioners to take the initiative to raise the topic of advance care planning, but also, to revisit directives once they have been drafted. By prompting health care providers to raise this issue and to not allow directives to lie stagnant, many of the problems[12] discussed earlier that arise with regard to advance care planning would be addressed.

However, while prompting health care providers to address the issue of advance care planning can be quite beneficial, certain provisos must accompany this directive. To instruct health care providers to address the topic of advance care planning as though it was tantamount to telling health care providers to remember to introduce themselves would be irresponsible. The notion that it is acceptable to simply start right in on advance care planning discussions is based in part on a false presupposition—that it is acceptable to discuss issues of death and dying directly. It is the lack of foundation for this presupposition that serves as the impetus for this book. If this "idealized" process is to be helpful in a culturally diverse setting, such false presuppositions need to be dispelled. If this flaw with the tool is noted and any attempts to engage patients in advance care planning are broached carefully and with the utmost cultural sensitivity, allowing for the patient to decline or, instead, to control which route the conversation takes, then the tool can serve as a nice prompt for health care providers engaging in advance care planning.

While there are tools offered in the Oncotalk learning guide that are useful at a very general level in terms of improving patient-provider communication, there are also suggestions that are particular to advance care planning. For example, the authors include a helpful reminder to providers to explore the "why" behind a patient's preference and to make sure that patient and provider have a shared understanding of the patient's goals (Fryer-Edwards et al. 2002, Module 4). This is extremely important in understanding what can be very vague instructions in a living will, for example. Specifically, in determining whether a patient would have wanted a certain treatment modality initiated, one can refer to the patient's goals and discern whether the treatments will serve to achieve such goals. If they will then there is strong evidence that the patient would have wanted treatments started. If not, then there is good evidence that the patient would have refused the treatments and thus, that these particular treatments should not be initiated.

Another benefit of Oncotalk is that it makes it clear that providers are offering patients an *opportunity* to discuss preferences for treatment and a chance to elucidate the values that ought to guide care at the end of life, not "forcing" patients to "give up," or forcing them to take advantage of the opportunity with which they are presented (Fryer-Edwards et al. 2002, Module 4). Emphasis is placed on letting patients know that such conversations are initiated with every patient in order to determine how best to establish and achieve goals set by the patient. Setting out advance care planning as a routine part of good care can help to alleviate anxiety that may arise when providers begin to talk about the intimate, often foreign issues that are involved in advance care planning. Similarly, the model reminds providers to focus not only on establishing the goals of the patient, but also, to "talk about the positive things that [the provider] can do to help the patient accomplish [her] future goals" (Fryer-Edwards et al. 2002, Module 4). This offers patients a bit of solace by reinforcing the measures health care providers can and will take to help patients reach their goals. By offering health care providers various "phrases that might be helpful" in engaging in the advance care planning process, the authors help providers get these difficult conversations started on the right path. Examples of such phrases include, "as you think about the illness, what is the best and worst that might happen?" "Have you seen or been with someone who had a particularly good death or a particularly bad death?" (Fryer-Edwards et al. 2002, Module 4). These questions help providers identify crucial issues, such as the patient's biggest fears about the illness. As was pointed out with the Kleinman model, knowing what is driving the patient's fears can help providers focus on alleviating specific worries. For instance, if the patient's biggest concern is dying in the hospital, providers can work on a treatment plan that includes care that would not necessitate a stay in the hospital (e.g., home hospice care). Addressing these worries can allow patients and families to focus on other issues and, hopefully, give them the opportunity to enjoy what time they have left together. Another benefit of these questions is that they help patients and families get specific. Inviting patients to think about particular cases of "good" and "bad" deaths allows them to paint a picture of situations that are and are not acceptable. Asking patients for stories of death and illness from their own experiences avoids the criticism often waged against advance directives of having to develop treatment preferences in a vacuum. Such specificity lies in stark contrast to simply asking patients what treatments they would and would not want if their "prognosis is poor." One area of particular note is Oncotalk's reminder to providers to thank patients and families for elucidating treatment preferences and goals of care and allowing the provider to share in what are usually very intimate details of the patient's life—a privileged view into one's conception of a good life. Suggestions for "closing" the conversation include things like, "'I want to thank you for helping me understand your values and goals'" (Fryer-Edwards et al. 2002, Module 4). At the end of the day, the patient has offered something of value to the provider, and as such, ought to be thanked.

For the most part, Oncotalk provides wonderful guidance for health care providers engaging in advance care planning. However, in discussing "theoretical considerations in DNR conversations," the suggestions offered in Oncotalk are prone to the criticism driving the call for increased culturally sensitivity—they have been developed out of the biomedical model and represent a very Western approach to advance care planning. For instance, while providers are encouraged to probe patients for explanations as to why certain treatment preferences have been chosen, and not simply leave patients to check "yes" or "no," some of the examples of how exactly to prompt the patient for further explanation are liable to cause harm to patients from certain cultures. In particular, when discussing how to get patients to elaborate a preference for CPR, one of the prompts given to health care providers is to ask, "What if something horrible happened and you had a stroke and I never thought you were going to wake up? Would you still want 'X'?" (Fryer-Edwards et al. 2002, Module 4). The model then has the health care provider delve further, asking the patient why he has requested or rejected the treatment at issue. However, by couching the question in terms of a hypothetical in which the patient himself is quite ill, the provider may have offended—indeed harmed—the patient. If that patient was a Navajo Indian who subscribed to the belief that simply voicing the potential for illness to befall an individual is to cause such an event to occur, this way of discussing advance care planning would be a grave mistake. To be sure, if the patient in question does not hold to the belief that words have the power to cause illness, such a way of approaching advance care planning (specifically decisions concerning CPR) could prove to be of great value. In the face of uncertainty though, one cannot take a chance and alternative approaches that are more culturally sensitive should be employed.

Voltz et al., in their Checklist for Planning of End-of-Life Decisions in Patients with a Terminal Disease, provide a great tool to prompt health care providers to ask some very basic, very important questions (Voltz et al. 1998). Questions on the checklist touch on issues such as where the patient would prefer to receive care (e.g., at home or in a hospital), determining how the patient is coping and whether further support is desired,[13] going over specific medical treatments with the patient to determine his preferences (e.g., CPR, respirators, artificial nutrition and hydration), all the way to whether the patient needs help with planning funeral details[14] (Voltz et al. 1998, 161). After going over "What should be discussed," the authors also include prompts for providers on "How to proceed if the patient wishes to express preferences in advance" (e.g., written and/or oral advance directives) (Voltz et al. 1998, 161–62). These prompts are appropriate, given that a central theme coming out of their paper is the idea that "an instrument to aid physicians, especially those not trained in palliative care, in planning for end-of-life decisions might be useful" (Voltz et al. 1998, 159). One interesting thing about this conclusion is the fact that it was drawn from research done in the United States, Germany, and Japan. It was an international study conducted in countries, some of which did not even have legislation recognizing advance directives and where advance directives were not given a warm welcome, and *still* aids for engaging in advance care planning were seen as useful, and not, as could have been the case, viewed as a waste of time and resources.

Further benefits of the checklist include the fact that it asks open-ended questions, leaving room for patients to explain their preferences and values to health care providers. However, that is but one edge of a double-edged sword. That the checklist offers prompts is good, but often times the stuff of advance care planning is foreign, unfamiliar territory on which patients need a good amount of guidance. If health care providers are not skilled in engaging patients in the advance care planning process, they may find themselves at a loss when patients don't take the initiative to expound on their preferences even after being prompted. Such a skill may be aided by more explicit direction, but it is certainly honed through practice. The hope is that in using the checklist providers find their footing, establish a rhythm, and do so without harming or offending their patients. In practice, this tool can be combined with some of the Oncotalk questions that really do well to direct patients to provide more specific direction and flesh out general preferences regarding treatment at the end of life.

A CASE FOR GREATER FAMILIAL
INVOLVEMENT IN ADVANCE CARE PLANNING

A useful strategy for engaging in advance care planning with individuals who prefer to involve family members, especially extended family, in the decision-making process is to encourage participation from family members at the outset. Involving family members in discussions surrounding such important decisions is not an uncommon preference, but in some cultures the input from family is weighted more heavily than even that of the patient. Chan provides an eloquent explanation of the role of the family in decision making in a more traditional biomedical view as opposed to a more robust conception of familial involvement, typical to various forms of "care ethics." He claims that in the biomedical model, the family has a role, indeed an important role in medical decision making, though such a role is "still inadequate because the family only serves to assist the incompetent patient to exercise her self-determination or to promote her individual interests. The model is entirely patient-centered, and the role of the family is marginalised in the sense of being subordinated to the choice and interests of the patient. The family becomes a shadow of the patient with no independent status and is therefore deprived of its self-sufficiency" (Chan 2004, 96). While certainly able to call upon her family for help, the patient is more than simply one voice amongst many. She has the ultimate authority to make medical decisions. Her family members may or may not concur. Ultimately, in the biomedical model, decision-making authority rests with the patient and it is up to the patient to determine whether she will make decisions in concert with family or go against familial prescriptions. In contrast, in the familial model "the role of the family is fundamental. . . . The interests of other family members are regarded as *inseparable* from my interests of the self" (Chan 2004, 96–98). Rather than having a lead vocalist (the patient) with a group of backup vocalists (family), as would be the case on the biomedical model when family joins with patient in making decisions, the familial model is more akin to a chorus of voices where no voice stands out, nor is any one voice more fundamental than another.

This practice of placing a strong emphasis on familial input and elevating familial needs above those of the individual can be seen clearly in the Hispanic value of *Familismo*. *Familismo* can be understood as "a collective loyalty to the extended family that outranks the needs of the individual. Important decisions are made by the family, not the individual alone" (Flores 2000, 16). A good way to respect individuals who place a great deal of importance on *Familismo* is to facilitate ways in which family members can get involved in the decision-making process. For example, with permission of the patient,[15] family members can be invited into the room to participate in the advance care planning process. Even though family members are present at the table for the discussions, the patient would be looked to for the final say — which may simply be an echoing of what the family has determined. Being proactive and inviting the patient to have his family with him, "providing ample time and opportunity for the extended family to gather to discuss important medical decisions," are all ways of showing respect and concern for a patient's cultural practices (Flores 2000, 16). During advance care planning, when the stakes are high and the tensions are equally as intense, any methods by which health care providers can decrease the likelihood that patients will feel insulted and increase the likelihood that patients will feel as though their ways of living have been respected[16] should be welcomed and lauded.

Following this line of thought on expanding the role of the family in the medical decision-making process, Chan has cleared the way for a co-starring role for family members in drafting advance directives. Chan has also forwarded a whole new way of operationalizing the instructions included in an advance directive. While an extensive examination of Chan's new "familial advance directive" will not be offered,[17] I want to highlight the perspective Chan offers on advance directives that could allow for them to be broached and completed with more success among populations that understand the family rather than the individual as the decision-making unit (Chan 2004, 96–98). Chan contrasts current advance directives (which he calls "individualistic advance directives") with "familial advance directives," maintaining that the latter provide several benefits for dealing with individuals from cultures where families are vested with decision-making power. Chan describes familial advance directives and some of their benefits as follows:

Instead of being a means for the patient to express her individual wish, an advance directive can be signed by the patient together with her family members so that they can communicate the wish of the family as a whole to the attending healthcare team. That can help reduce the possible conflicts between family members and the healthcare team when the patient becomes incompetent. [In addition] the introduction of familial advance directives can serve to trigger off more sharing discussions about advance care planning among family members, including the patient, and facilitate better communication among them. (Chan 2004, 97)

Given this conception of an advance directive, an important role for the family is not only permitted or tolerated, but such a role is welcomed. With the familial advance directive, from the outset, the family is included in the advance care planning process as a matter of protocol rather than as a matter of accommodating the whim of the patient. Such inclusionary practices can make the patient more comfortable and allow for a relationship to be established between health care providers and families that may not have had a chance to evolve given the fast-paced clinical setting. Having a relationship and being able to negotiate an understanding prior to a patient becoming incompetent can prove to be invaluable after a patient is no longer able to speak for himself. Any ambiguities from patient, provider, and/or family members can be brought out and clarified while the patient is still able to maintain an active voice in the medical treatment plan. So too, establishing such relationships allows for patients and families to become familiar with how the health care provider(s) handle medical treatment and decision making, and vice-versa. This familiarity can serve as a solid foundation on which to build consensus if the patient becomes incompetent.

Chan does acknowledge that there may be a case (here Chan gives the example of a dysfunctional family) in which the "fundamental interests of the patient" are at risk of being abused (Chan, 2004, 102). In such cases,

the physician should follow the familial practice unless the patient has shown her disapproval in the first place. This provides leeway for the patient to safeguard herself from abuse and neglect. However, the burden of disapproval is on those who want to veto the practice. So the physician does not need to clarify this with the patient in the first place; it is the patient's responsibility to let the physician know the objection beforehand. If the patient does not do that, the physician will not be charged with malpractice. (Chan 2004, 102)

While this option for "opting out" does provide the patient with some means of protection, given that it is the "fundamental interests" of the patient that are at issue, one is lead to wonder whether such "protection" is sufficient. For instance, rather than having the onus of disapproval of the familial model rest with the patient, instead, it should be an obligation on the part of the provider to ask the patient whether or not she approves of employing the familial model. Shifting the responsibility for determining the appropriateness of the familial model from the patient to the physician is fitting given that the patient is already sick and in fact may be unfamiliar with the need to "opt out" in the first place. Chan's model can be improved with this shift in responsibility without infringing on the integral role for family in the medical decision-making process.

No matter the cultural perspective at issue, during advance care planning it is important to focus on the goals rather than specific treatments.[18] This will help to contextualize the preferences of the patient. If providers focus on asking whether or not patients want or refuse particular treatments, patients will most likely give "yes" or "no" responses. Conversely, when inviting patients to make decisions based on their goals, what it is that they deem most important, what makes a life worth living, more detail will need to be provided in order to convey the message. This will furnish provider and patient with the opportunities to ask questions, gain greater insight into the nuances surrounding a patient's preferences, participate in a conversation rather than a one-way series of questions, and help to foster a trusting relationship. As Quill notes, "Trust is fostered when physicians try to learn about each patient's and family's unique story and then share their own medical expertise and recommendations in ways that respect that history and experience which is both culturally defined and unique" (Quill 2002, 232). Overall, any model aimed at helping health care providers engage in culturally sensitive advance care planning is limited by the level of participation of the patient. Tools such as those listed above are quite useful at pointing out general issues with which providers ought to be aware, but it is the patient and the patient's family who bring to the table the other crucial component—information about the particular patient and how the general issues do and do not apply to her. Information at both the general and specific levels is necessary for successful advance care planning.

One area where patients and families can offer invaluable information is with regard to the traditional health practices in which they engage. If the patient and the health care provider have a good relationship, where patient and family feel comfortable telling the provider about some of their traditional health practices, being aware of such practices could facilitate a more active role for patient and family in the care plan. Incorporating traditional health practices is one way to tailor treatment for an individual at the end of life and get patients, families, and providers working from a common understanding. While health care providers should never underestimate the importance of incorporating traditional practices alongside "modern" medicine, not knowing about a patient's use of traditional health care practices poses even greater dangers than a limited conception of acceptable treatment options. Transparency about the care a patient is receiving would allow for the health care practitioner to investigate any of the traditional remedies that the patient and family might be using in order to determine if there are any contraindications. Thus, patient safety would be increased by minimizing the risk of serious complications that might arise if the patient and family used such remedies unbeknownst to the health care team. Hence, the benefits of building a trusting relationship between patient and provider go beyond establishing open lines of communication (though this is clearly a critical component of a successful provider-patient relationship), to include minimizing the risk of adverse events in the course of caring for a patient. One of the keys to achieving such trust and reaping these benefits is being "culturally aware"[19] and interacting with patients in a culturally sensitive manner.

NEXT STEPS: CULTURALLY SENSITIVE EDUCATION

Education on how to provide culturally sensitive care must be established as a primary component in training health care providers. Incorporating such training into the various health care curricula can be facilitated if such a change is backed by various agencies and governing bodies within the health care domain. For example, The United States Department of Health and Human Services, through the Office of Minority Health, has developed "standards for cultural and linguistically appropriate health care services" (CLAS standards).[20] Broken down into three themes, Culturally Competent Care, Language Access Services, and Organizational Supports for Cultural Competence, these standards are then further sorted into varying degrees of stringency: mandates, guidelines, and recommendations (www.hhs.gov, accessed January 21, 2009). Though geared toward guidance on the organizational level, the CLAS standards are also useful at the level of the individual provider. Under the theme "Culturally Competent Care" are the first three standards, all of which are guidelines that are "recommended by the Office of Minority Health for adoption as mandates by Federal, State, and national accrediting agencies" (www.hhs.gov, accessed January 21, 2009):

Standard 1

Health care organizations should ensure that patients/consumers receive from all staff members effective, understandable, and respectful care that is provided in a manner compatible with their cultural health beliefs and practices and preferred language.

Standard 2

Health care organizations should implement strategies to recruit, retain, and promote at all levels of the organization a diverse staff and leadership that are representative of the demographic characteristics of the service area.

Standard 3

Health care organizations should ensure that staff at all levels and across all disciplines receive ongoing education and training in culturally and linguistically appropriate service delivery.

Standards 1 through 3 serve to highlight the importance of communicating in a culturally sensitive manner, recruiting a diverse staff that reflects the population served by the institution, and the need for continuing education for staff on how to foster and increase the level of cultural sensitivity throughout the organization. It is by combining efforts with the goal of excelling in all of these areas that an organization will increase its level of cultural sensitivity. That the CLAS standards were developed at a national level, "based on an analytical review of key laws, regulations, contracts, and standards currently in use by federal and state agencies and other national organizations," gives them an authority derived from the broad, rich research that went into their creation (Spector 2003, 7). Such a solid foundation on which to base the call for an increase in culturally sensitive health care is a wonderful starting point to promote widespread change.

In addition, "The Liason Committee on Medical Education (LCME) states in their accreditation standards that 'The faculty and students must demonstrate an understanding of the manner in which people of diverse cultures and belief systems perceive health and illness and respond to various symptoms, diseases, and treatments'" (Crandall et al. 2003, 588). Not only does the LCME call for medical students to understand the belief systems of others, but also, to "recognize and appropriately address gender and cultural bias in themselves and others, and in the process of health care delivery" (Crandall et al. 2003, 588). Incorporating these requirements into accreditation standards serves to reinforce the importance of achieving high levels of cultural sensitivity. By formalizing the call for increasing cultural sensitivity in the delivery of health care, such a goal is no longer an added benefit patients would be lucky to happen upon with some providers. Rather, it is a threshold under which health care providers ought not to fall. In listing the growing number of professional associations and accrediting bodies that are incorporating cultural competence into their standards and guidelines, Crandall et al. note the following:

> The American Medical Student Association's Promoting, Reinforcing and Improving Medical Education project (AMSA PRIME) has solicited requests for proposals from schools to pilot a cultural competency curriculum using the association's established core competencies. The Accreditation Council of Graduate Medical Education and the Council on Graduate Medical Education are increasingly emphasizing the importance of cultural competency. . . . Guidelines and competencies have already appeared for residency programs. The National Board of Medical Examiners will ultimately focus on cultural competency skill as one requirement for passing licensing exams. (Crandall et al. 2003, 588–89)

For several decades, nursing associations and professional organizations have recognized the importance of incorporating "cultural content" in nursing education programs. For example, "As early as 1977, the National League for Nursing required cultural content in nursing curricula and in 1991, the American Nursing Association published standards specifically indicating that culturally and ethnically relevant care should be available to all patients" (Smedley et al. 2002, 203).

CULTURALLY SENSITIVE EDUCATIONAL MATERIALS

Not only must the education of health care providers have as a goal the provision of culturally sensitive care, the educational materials that are available to patients and families must also be culturally sensitive. Armed with culturally sensitive educational materials, health care providers stand a better chance of broaching highly charged topics (like advance care planning) within a pluralistic clinical setting without creating conflict. Regardless of how much or how little information is requested by the patient, the educational materials, both extant and forthcoming, need to convey information in a culturally sensitive way. The National Cancer Alliance is spot on in its request for educational materials to be developed that are culturally sensitive, "Culturally sensitive patient information materials need to be produced, which make partnership between health care professionals and patients a reality by offering support for people to really own and embed their illness in the context of what already makes sense to them (National Cancer Alliance, as cited in Mystakidou et al. 2005, 180).

Determining where culturally sensitive materials need to be developed may sound like a daunting task. There are so many places that such material would be beneficial, yet resources are limited. Patient populations can be so diverse and one's own capabilities limited at best in terms of developing culturally sensitive educational materials. In attempting to address such limitations, providers and institutions need to identify which educational materials are given to patients most frequently. This will help to ensure that resources are spent on materials that are distributed widely, as opposed to materials that are rarely used. Institutions have such distribution data that they can mine in order to identify those areas where making educational materials culturally sensitive could reach large sections of the various patient populations at issue. So too, by determining the demographic of one's patient population, various materials that are displayed in patient areas (e.g., waiting or exam rooms) can be translated into representative languages. With regard to advance care planning, materials created to facilitate the process of advance care planning need to be available in several languages. If a patient requests such material in a language not readily available, health care providers need to be able to access someone or some institution that could provide translating services. Clearly, advance directives ought to be available in appropriate languages for the larger patient populations served by an institution, and interpreting services should be available to patients who want to discuss issues surrounding such directives in more detail with providers.

Another method of increasing the amount of culturally sensitive materials is through both the institutional intranet and the internet. With regard to the intranet, by placing links to overviews on cultural issues in the clinical setting and useful websites,[21] health care providers would have easy access to information that can help them gain an understanding of some issues they may be facing. Other useful links for providers would be to community groups representative of the patient populations for which they care.[22] In addition to placing external links to community groups, contact information for the person or department in charge of cultural competency education should also be posted so that providers who need additional information know where to turn within the institution. Links for such resources ought to be placed prominently and labeled clearly on the intranet so that providers have as little difficulty as possible accessing this crucial information. Prominent placement may also serve to give such resources more "visibility" within the institution and increase awareness of the importance of education on providing culturally sensitive care. Overall, the capacity to educate patients and successfully convey complex medical information is a fundamental component in providing health care, and becoming culturally sensitive is critical to such an endeavor. Thus, in striving to communicate with patients more successfully, health care providers must pay close attention to increasing their level of cultural sensitivity and to making educational tools more accessible to a diverse patient population.

When an institution engages in developing its own educational programs and resources, any tools that are developed can and should be tailored to the particular demographic served by the institution. One way to increase the likelihood that institutional programs are meeting the needs of the patient populations at issue, as was mentioned earlier, is by inviting participation from the communities served by the institution. Investing time and energy into creating an inclusive group composed of community leaders from the patient populations served by the institution that can engage health care providers and community members in a discourse will prove to be an invaluable short and long term venture. "Community informants" and "cultural liaisons" are some of the other names by which these community members are known (James 2005). James describes a cultural liaison as "someone who is active in the community, understands [the health care provider's] concerns and introduces [health care providers] to the people [in the community] who can make a difference" (James 2005, 26). In the short term, information can be gained directly from these "cultural liaisons" on how to better approach patients from various backgrounds. By enlisting the help of community leaders it is more likely that members of the community will be forthcoming and engage in a meaningful dialogue. Long-term dividends of establishing ties to community leaders include having at your disposal a list of well-connected, well-respected individuals upon whom you can call for insight into cultural issues. In addition, such contacts in the community can also be useful resources for educational activities. For example, in order to educate staff about various cultural perspectives on dealing with illness within a particular cultural group, community leaders can be called upon to give talks and provide in-services. These educational events are illuminating on a number of different levels. Such talks not only help health care providers gain an understanding of how people from different cultural backgrounds perceive and deal with illness, but they also help community leaders understand the misconceptions that may exist on the part of health care providers. Community leaders can answer questions from health care providers and also take away with them an understanding of where the health care providers are coming from in their attempt to care for patients. For instance, if a conflict arises out of a cultural misunderstanding between providers and members from the community a given leader represents, the leader may be able to help out by recognizing where the misconception *on both sides* resides and help to facilitate an accord.

In short, seeking out and fostering relationships with well-respected community leaders helps health care providers and institutions gain "buy-in" or "credibility" within a given community, provides options for individuals on whom to call to take part in educational activities in the health care institution, and can help to convey the overall message that when cultural conflicts arise, they are not necessarily born out of an unwillingness to accommodate different practices, but rather out of a misunderstanding and a lack of awareness. Even if this sentiment of community involvement and exerted efforts to gain a better understanding of the cultural issues that exist in the community has been put out by the institution in the past, greater credence might be given to it when voiced by a community leader on behalf of the institution. By harnessing the knowledge and insight that exist right outside its front door, through establishing relationships with community members, an institution can stay up-to-date on current attitudes and views that might influence how medical care is perceived.

Valuable resources can also be found within the institution. Calling on and consulting with colleagues from different cultures is a great way to tap into a ready-made knowledge base without even having to leave the building. Consulting with culturally diverse colleagues will provide an opportunity to identify conflicts in the early stages—hopefully helping to discharge them before they erupt. Tapping into such resources entails having the resources within the institution in the first place. Institutions can ensure that these valuable resources are available by hiring and recruiting culturally diverse health care providers, specifically those representative of the patient populations served. Wright et al. suggest some useful strategies for providers and institutions working to increase the level of cultural sensitivity with which health care is provided:

> Strategies include having written resources available on each unit, designing events to highlight individual groups, celebrating culturally sensitive holidays, and designating staff who can provide individual information on a formal or informal basis. Inviting families of patients who have been discharged. . . . To return to staff meetings and discuss how the staff can be more culturally sensitive, although potentially uncomfortable for staff, is an excellent way to open up discussion and dialogue. (Wright et al. 1997, 72)

Another way to gain insight from patients and families would be to have them meet with the bioethicist, or a member from the ethics committee if there is no bioethicist on staff at the hospital. This more intimate meeting can help to make patient and family more comfortable opening up about their experiences and offering constructive criticism. The bioethicist would then be charged with the task of compiling the results from the meeting and offering them to the health care team and discussing ways in which this data could improve patient care in the future. Insights obtained from these meetings can be relayed to several units via in-services and even posted on the intranet for future reference by staff.

An interesting and simple suggestion on how providers can increase their understanding and familiarity with the patient populations they serve is to become more familiar with the daily activities and traditions of other cultures. For instance, health care providers can attend cultural events sponsored by various cultural groups in the area. Whether it be through inviting cultural leaders in the community to give talks, holding potluck dinners[23] for staff that focus on different cultures, or by exploring various shops and restaurants in the community where high concentrations of individuals from different cultures go, simply by engaging in, organizing, and highlighting the importance of events, greater awareness of other cultures is achieved. Awareness is the first step in reaching the goal of providing culturally sensitive care. As James explains, "Interaction focused on learning about other cultures . . . and hopefully one's own, helps to 'promote culturally sensitive minds'" (James 2005, 26).

ENHANCING CULTURAL SENSITIVITY THROUGHOUT THE ORGANIZATION

Cultural sensitivity must be a goal that is cultivated at all levels of an organization. Its importance and an emphasis on supporting programs and policies that focus on it cannot be overemphasized. Organizations must aim toward ensuring that patients are met with individuals in the health care organization that are culturally sensitive. Such a standard is "relevant not only to staff, who ultimately are responsible for the kinds of interactions they have with patients, but also to their organizations, which must provide the managers, policies, and systems that support the realities of culturally competent[24] encounters" (Bronheim and Sockalingam 2003, 7). That is, the goal of achieving cultural sensitivity throughout an organization cannot be realized unless it is viewed as an integral part of the vision and values of the health care organization. Health care providers seeking to increase their level of cultural sensitivity would be hard-pressed to do so in an institution that did not give such a goal any weight. Having policies and procedures to refer to, having champions of cultural sensitivity at all levels of the organization, having the provision of culturally sensitive care as a core value of the organization—these are things that are invaluable in creating a culturally competent organization. More specifically, cultural competence requirements have been developed for organizations.

Cultural competence[25] requires that organizations:

- Have a defined set of values and principles, and demonstrate behaviors, attitudes, policies, and structures that enable them to work effectively cross-culturally.
- Have the capacity to (1) value diversity, (2) conduct self-assessment, (3) manage the dynamics of difference, (4) acquire and institutionalize

cultural knowledge, and (5) adapt to diversity and the cultural contexts of the communities they serve.
- Incorporate the above in all aspects of policy making, administration, practice/service delivery and systematically involve consumers/families. (Bronheim and Sockalingam 2003, 2)

Given the importance of practicing culturally sensitive health care, it is imperative that some direction be provided to organizations to begin developing policies and programs focused on achieving this goal. Programs aimed at fostering cultural sensitivity within the organization should not be developed in a vacuum. Rather, they ought to be informed by the patient population they serve. There would need to be general guidelines put in place, but specific programs should be developed that target some of the larger patient populations served by the institution. Developing these targeted programs makes sense on many levels. By focusing efforts to increase cultural sensitivity, an organization can be more economical in terms of time spent on development of programs, and at the same time, the programs developed will be more efficient, as efforts will be concentrated on the very populations that are served most frequently by the organization.

How, then, can an organization go about focusing such efforts? One of the first steps would be to develop a sort of needs assessment of some of the main patient populations that focuses on cultural issues. Not only would this help to identify some of the key cultural beliefs and practices at issue, but it also helps get the community involved in a plan that has helping them as one of its main goals. Including the community from the outset will also help to create a relationship between the organization and the members of the community built on mutual respect and a willingness to listen to ideas generated from all parties. In other words, the community will gain buy-in to the programs that are developed, and at the end of the development process community members can feel as if they were a part of the final product. Community members will have been given an opportunity to be heard and their values and beliefs woven into the fabric of programs established to foster cultural sensitivity. The importance of emphasizing cultural sensitivity throughout the organization makes sense. It is not only physicians and nurses that patients and families come into contact with when they enter into a health care institution. A bad experience with anyone from a maintenance worker to an administrator can sour a patient and family to the health care institution as a whole.[26]

In an effort to increase the level of cultural competence of health care institutions, The National Center for Cultural Competence at Georgetown University has developed a list of actions and behaviors that culturally competent organizations[27] need to implement[28]:

- Create a missions statement for the organization that articulates principles, rationale, and values for cultural and linguistic competence in all aspects of the organization.
- Implement specific policies and procedures that integrate cultural and linguistic competence into each core function of the organization.
- Identify, use, and/or adapt evidence-based and promising practices that are culturally and linguistically competent.
- Develop structures and strategies to ensure consumer and community participation in the planning, delivery, and evaluation of the organization's core function.
- Implement policies and procedures to recruit, hire, and maintain a diverse and culturally and linguistically competent workforce.
- Provide fiscal support, professional development, and incentives for the improvement of cultural and linguistic competence at the board, program, and faculty and/or staff levels.
- Dedicate resources for both individual and organizational self-assessment of cultural and linguistic competence.
- Develop the capacity to collect and analyze data using variables that have meaningful impact on culturally and linguistically diverse groups.
- Practice principles of community engagement that result in the reciprocal transfer of knowledge and skills between all collaborators, partners, and key stakeholders. (A Guide to Infusing Cultural & Linguistic Competence in Health Promotion Training: Group Activity—Understanding the Cultural Competence Continuum 4, accessed November 2006).

Going even further, The National Center for Cultural Competence describes a health care organization that has reached the ultimate in cultural competence—"cultural proficiency." This is one "level" above being a culturally competent organization. All of the aforementioned actions and behaviors are still applicable, however, a culturally proficient organization does not just manifest "an acceptance and respect for cultural differences," it "holds culture in high esteem" and integrates culture as a pivotal part of the foundation guiding all of its "endeavors" (A Guide to Infusing Cultural & Linguistic Competence in Health Promotion Training: Group Activity—Understanding the Cultural Competence Continuum 4–5, accessed November 2006). Striking to note about a culturally proficient organization is that it not only goes to great lengths to increase the level of cultural competence of existing faculty/staff, but also it sets out to hire new staff members that are experts in cultural competence education and research. This commitment to increase cultural competence is manifested not only in the hiring practices of culturally proficient organizations, but also in such an organization's dedication to "advocating" for both unserved and underserved populations, and on concentrating efforts on reducing and eliminating many of the "racial and ethnic disparities" that occur in the populations that they serve (A Guide to Infusing Cultural & Linguistic Competence in Health Promotion Training: Group Activity—Understanding the Cultural Competence Continuum 5, accessed November 2006). Overall, it is no small feat to become a culturally competent organization. Even institutions that achieve this goal still have room to aspire to attaining culturally proficient status.

The call for increasing cultural sensitivity is also clear at the level of health care organization accreditation. For example, The Joint Commission,[29] in their study, *Hospitals, Language, and Culture: A Snapshot of the Nation*, posed the following question to "physicians and nurses at 60 U.S. hospitals":

> Juan Lopez, a Hispanic man with limited English proficiency, is admitted to your hospital with severe abdominal pain. You think he needs surgery, but he insists that the pain is the result of a hex, and requests treatment from a witch doctor. How do you respond? (Butterfield 2008, accessed July 16, 2008)

That such a question was part of a study by the Joint Commission, the largest accrediting body for health care organizations in the United States, underscores the importance placed on providing culturally sensitive care.

Buttressing the efforts of organizations to become culturally sensitive, states have begun to require cultural competency training for physicians. While California and New Jersey are leading the way, other states are beginning to follow suit.

> *California.* Continuing medical education (CME) courses for California physicians will be required to contain curricula in cultural and linguistic competency beginning July 1, 2006. The new requirement is contained in Assembly Bill (A.B.) 1195 signed by Governor Arnold Schwazenegger on October 4. Under A.B.1195, cultural and linguistic competency care will be a component of all continuing medical education courses, except for research or other courses that do not include direct patient care and courses offered by out-of-state CME providers. Accreditation associations for CME are required to develop standards for this curriculum before July 1, 2006. *New Jersey.* A more comprehensive bill was approved by New Jersey Acting Governor, Richard J. Codey, on March 23, 2005. The New Jersey bill (S.144) requires physician training in cultural competence in order to obtain a license from or to be re-licensed by the State Board of Medical Examiners. New Jersey licensed physicians will have to document that they have completed cultural competency training no later than March 23, 2008 (three years after the act's effective date) as a condition of relicensure.[30] (Butterfield 2008, accessed July 16, 2008)

Against such a strong backdrop of multi-level support, the setting is ideal for culturally sensitive care to gain residence as a fundamental component of providing quality health care.

ASSESSING EFFORTS TO INCREASE
CULTURAL COMPETENCY

The importance of gathering data on the success (or lack thereof) with which various interventions and strategies for increasing cultural sensitivity have been met cannot be overlooked. Such information will serve to better direct the development of future projects and policies aimed at increasing cultural sensitivity. In addition, if such endeavors are shown to increase cultural sensitivity, this information will help to strengthen the case for increased funding in this area. Ideally, increased cultural sensitivity will effectuate change not only in relationships between health care providers and patients, but also, in the relationships forged amongst health care providers. Raising awareness of the plurality of views that may be brought to the table should serve to facilitate a working environment in which the importance of mutual respect and understanding is underscored. Determining which strategies are most successful in creating such environments is a necessary part of any serious endeavor to increase cultural sensitivity.

Performing an overall needs assessment prior to implementing any strategies aimed at increasing cultural sensitivity is a good way to establish a baseline against which any changes can be measured. After establishing this baseline, gathering data from a needs assessment, and developing programs that address the needs identified, the success of the interventions can be measured in various ways. One way of measuring various methods is to administer a survey. To be sure, the population(s) receiving the survey will vary depending upon the specific questions that need to be addressed in a particular institution. Nonetheless, a good way to get a general sense of the efficacy of the changes and/or educational programs that were implemented is to administer a patient satisfaction survey. Focusing not only on the general level of patient satisfaction, but also looking at areas that would be directly influenced by programs targeted at increasing cultural sensitivity is a way to gain some insight into which direction future programs should go. For instance, questions could include whether access to interpreter services was gained with ease, whether the patients felt as though health care providers engaged them in discussions in a manner that respected their customs and beliefs, and also whether patients felt as though their interests and concerns were respected in their health care encounter. Overall, patient satisfaction surveys should, at least, try and determine how well patients felt that they were listened to in their encounter with health care providers. Prima facie, the notion of "being listened to" may seem to be quite broad. However, it does well to capture the spirit of any program aimed at increasing cultural sensitivity. Namely, a program wherein relationships are forged with the goal of respect for the concerns and interests of all parties, and appropriate weighing of the voices of those involved in the decision-making process.

Just as important as gauging the perceptions of patients and families is making sure that the perceptions of the staff have been taken into account as well. Surveys that assess the impact of interventions to increase cultural sensitivity from the perspective of the health care provider are a key component in determining the effectiveness of such measures. Provider surveys could help determine, for instance, if providers report fewer cultural conflicts, if they have been able to communicate with patients from different cultures better after receiving education on cross-cultural communication, and whether the level of cultural sensitivity has increased in the interactions between health care providers. Further, in order for the administration of the health care institution to gauge how well interventions are working amongst health care providers, anonymous "quizzes" could be distributed[31] to see if providers are aware of how to approach patients, families, and fellow workers in a culturally sensitive manner. Another way to make this determination is to observe clinical interactions between both provider and patient, and between providers. To be sure, this direct observation would be more informed if done by someone trained in cross-cultural communication strategies. Enlisting the help of such a person at the outset would make the most sense. Even more, hiring someone with the training to develop and implement a needs assessment, construct and deliver educational sessions based on the results of the needs assessment, and then evaluate the level of success of such projects would seem to be a wise investment that would pay tremendous dividends in terms of increased cultural competence and sensitivity. This individual could also continue to consult on an "as needed" basis as educational efforts are expanded and amended.

A good way for an institution to get the "most bang for the buck" is to have trained individuals train key people in the institution to be trainers themselves (i.e., train the trainers). The "trainers" within the institution can provide support and continue to strive toward the goal of increasing cultural competence and sensitivity. Such individuals would have a privileged perspective in that they are in the health care institution on a daily basis, familiar with the staff, and able to watch as the various strategies to increase cultural sensitivity are "rolled out." In addition, they can provide real time feedback as to how well (or not) various programs are working and what sort of response they are getting on various units. Overall, by having health care providers trained as trainers, an institution can better monitor and develop a culturally sensitive environment. Regardless of which assessment methodology is employed, it "should match the educational objectives and be carried out in a careful, step-wise fashion, controlling for all possible cofounders and focusing first on process measures (such as patient and provider satisfaction)" (Smedley et al. 2002, 203).

CONCLUSION: BE OPEN, BE AWARE

Engaging in advance care planning is a difficult, sensitive endeavor. This is true even when the people involved in the process share similar cultural beliefs and values. Since it is often the case that those involved in the advance care planning process enter into the relationship with different values and, sometimes, entirely different worldviews, providing a space for everyone to meet and share their varied perspectives, rather than coming to the table with a pre-established notion of what a "good" result would be, is central to the success of the process. Health care providers need to be open to the possibility that there are several ways to achieve the goal of doing what is "best for the patient." Even more than simply allowing for the possibility of differences, providing culturally sensitive care requires providers to actively engage a patient to help understand who the patient is (Spector 2003, 302). The tools that I have included in this book serve as nice examples of how to help health care providers strive to understand their patients, how best to work through emotionally charged discussions, and overall, effectively communicate cross-culturally. Achieving these goals requires that health care providers understand that it is their duty, as part of providing culturally sensitive care, to try and understand the perspectives from which their patients are coming and engage with them at a level that everyone deems acceptable. While the various cross-cultural communication tools can help providers begin to open a dialogue with patients and families, it is the overall attitude of the providers and the environment in the institution itself on which the drive to provide culturally sensitive care will stand or fall. Setting out to become a culturally sensitive institution needs to be a central part of the vision of the health care institution.

Implementing various educational programs and making use of the cultural resources both inside and outside of the institution will be a key factor in realizing this vision. Health care providers can also rely on resources such as a bioethicist, cultural leaders in the community, health care providers from various cultures, and hospital librarians. Too often the valuable insight to be gained by simply asking those right next to you is overlooked. Such considerations are on the radar of a culturally sensitive provider. Ultimately, providing culturally sensitive care is achieved not by wrote memorization of a cornucopia of cultural beliefs and practices. Rather, it is evidenced in the greater awareness providers have of the complexity of providing health care in a multicultural setting, in the accommodations made to facilitate good communication with patients no matter their background, by the ties the health care institution has established with cultural leaders and community members in general, and, most importantly, by the high level of satisfaction patients have in their health care encounters. Proceeding with caution, a spirit of inquiry, and a willingness to deviate from the norm is the best plan for successful interactions in the increasingly diverse health care context.

NOTES

1. See Freedman in Steinbock et al. 2008.

2. This information can be found at The National Center for Health Statistics (www.cdc.gov/nchs/Default.htm). For additional useful sites, see *A Guide to Infusing Cultural & Linguistic Competence in Health Promotion Training*, National Center for Cultural Competence, Georgetown University Center for Child & Human Development (pp. 1–2: Group Activity—Who Lives in Our Area?).

3. This information is available at The Migration Information Source (migrationinformation.org.USFocus/statemap.cfm). For additional useful sites, see *A Guide to Infusing Cultural & Linguistic Competence in Health Promotion Training*, National Center for Cultural Competence, Georgetown University Center for Child & Human Development (pp. 1–2: Group Activity—Who Lives in Our Area?).

4. Oncotalk is a training program for oncology fellows, funded in part by The Greenwall Foundation and by the National Cancer Institute. The website for the Oncotalk program is: depts.washington.edu/oncotalk/. The information I draw on comes from the manual, "Tough Talk: Helping Doctors Approach Difficult Conversations, A Toolbox For Medical Educators," obtained at the ASBH Pre-Course October 2004. More information can be found at the Oncotalk website.

5. Werth et al. explain this compilation of approaches to culturally sensitive communication as follows: "Several authors have offered guidelines in an effort to help make end-of-life care more culturally sensitive (e.g., Hallenbeck and Goldstein 1999; B. A. Koenig and Gates-Williams 1995). Ersek and colleagues (1998; see p.1687) modified B. A. Koenig and Gates-Williams's (1995) guidelines (see Kagawa-Singer and Blackhall 2001, for a different modification) and provided the following suggestions for assessing cultural variations in end-of-life situations" (Werth et al. 214)

6. For a full account of Leininger's model, see Leininger and McFarland 2006.

7. Thanks to Kerry Bowman for clarifying this point.

8. Some examples of such resources are community leaders, colleagues from different cultural groups, community health workers, and bioethicists who can help to facilitate communication between patients and providers, and can help gather resources and develop in-services focused on increasing cultural sensitivity.

9. Koenig does well to capture some of these values when describing "the 'American mainstream values' that affect nursing interactions when approaching end-of-life decisions. These values include the beliefs that (1) the competent adult patient should make his or her own decisions; (2) individualism not collectivism, is the norm; (3) informing the patient of the diagnosis and prognosis is a universal moral good regardless of eventual expected outcome; (4) open candid discussion of end-of-life decisions is universally desirable" (Koenig, as cited in Wright et al. 1997, 64–65).

10. In this case, the "Africentric cultural belief system of ancestors and spirits" is at issue (Parry and Ryan 1995).

11. A complete list of questions and a more extensive analysis of the Giger-Davidhizar Model can be found in J. Giger and R. Davidhizar *Transcultural Nursing: Assessment and Intervention* (St. Louis: Mosby Year Book, 2004).

12. For instance, providers are prompted to begin the discussion on advance care planning rather than wait and see if the patient brings it up. Providers are also reminded to review and update advance directives. Updating directives not only serves to keep the preferences documented in them current by having to refer to them periodically, but also it helps with the very practical issue of making sure that patients and providers know where the directive is if it is needed.

13. Here different notions of "support" can be explored. For example, the clinical social worker may need to get involved to figure out how to secure additional home health services. So too, the patient may be concerned about support for his family and express a desire for counseling that would include his whole family and help everyone deal with his illness.

14. This could mean anything from putting family members in touch with local funeral homes, all the way to determining how best to respect a patient and family's wish to have the patient buried within a certain timeframe.

15. The patient would be asked whether or not he wanted to invite family members in to discuss advance care planning while he was alone with the health care provider. This way, the patient would not have to refuse entrance to family members when they were in the same room. This would also allow the patient to put the question off until a later time and allow him to think about the possible consequences of engaging in such discussions with his family members in the room.

16. Respected insofar as such different practices have been put forth, listened to, understood, and appreciated, and, where possible, incorporated into the treatment plan.

17. For a more complete account of Chan's "familial advance directive," see Chan 2004.

18. See chapter 1 where I discuss the benefits of goal-based as opposed to treatment-based advance directives.

19. Thanks to Ken Goodman for suggesting this term.

20. The Joint Commission 2008 Requirements Related to the Provision of Culturally and Linguistically Appropriate Health Care, April 2008. www.jointcommission.org/NR/rdonlyres/6941959E-D4BE-48D7-A2F8A4834E84B263/0/JC_Standards_Document_2008.pdf, accessed January 27, 2009.

21. Here an institution could place links to helpful articles and books on the subject. For a more ready-reference, some useful websites could be listed. For example:

The National Center for Cultural Competence at Georgetown University Center for Child and Human Development, www.nccccurricula.info/modules.html; The U.S. Department of Health and Human Services Office of Minority Health, www.omhrc. gov/; Joint Commission on Accreditation of Healthcare Organizations Hospitals, Language and Culture Project, www.jointcommission.org/HLC.

22. In order to get as much out of the links to the community groups, institutions should seek to establish relationships with the leaders of such groups, and ultimately, establish a sort of "point person" with whom to make first contact if needed. More will be said about establishing relationships with leaders of various community cultural groups in the next paragraph.

23. The idea for a "potluck dinner" comes from James 2005.

24. Here I am taking "cultural competence" to refer to the same thing as "cultural sensitivity."

25. Here again I understand a "culturally competent" organization to refer to the same thing as a "culturally sensitive" organization.

26. Multicultural Palliative Care Guidelines: Andrew Taylor and Margaret Box, Palliative Care Australia, 1999.

27. These actions and behaviors hold for both health care organizations and health care systems. Here again I understand a "culturally competent" organization to refer to the same thing as a "culturally sensitive" organization.

28. From "A Guide to Infusing Cultural & Linguistic Competence in Health Promotion Training: Group Activity-Understanding the Cultural Competence Continuum." National Center for Cultural Competence. www11.georgetown.edu/research/gucchd/nccc/projects/sids/dvd/continuum.pdf (p. 4).

29. The Joint Commission is "An independent, not-for-profit organization, The Joint Commission accredits and certifies more than 15,000 health care organizations and programs in the United States. Joint Commission accreditation and certification is recognized nationwide as a symbol of quality that reflects an organization's commitment to meeting certain performance standards" (www.jointcommission.org/AboutUs/, accessed July 17, 2008).

30. In addition, "New Jersey and Washington have also passed laws requiring cultural medical education, and legislation is pending in Illinois, New York and Ohio" (www.acponline.org/clinical_information/journals_publications/acp_hospitalist/mar08/cover.htm, accessed July 16, 2008).

31. Distribution could take place, for example, via email or after in-services focused on increasing cultural sensitivity.

References

Introduction

Berry, Scott R., and Peter A. Singer. "The Cancer Specific Advance Directive." *Cancer* 82, no. 8 (April 1998): 1570–77.

Butterfield, Stacey. "A Different Kind of Competency." *ACP Hospitalist*. 2008. www.acponline.org/clinical_information/journals_publications/acp_hospitalist/mar08/cover.htm (accessed July 17, 2008).

Cantor, Norman L. "Prospective Autonomy: On the Limits of Shaping One's Post-Competence Medical Fate." *Journal of Contemporary Health Law and Policy* 8 (Spring 1992):13–48.

———. *Advance Directives and the Pursuit of Death with Dignity*. Bloomington: Indiana University Press, 1993.

Crawley, LaVera M., Patricia A. Marshall, Bernard Lo, and Barbara A. Koenig. "Strategies for Culturally Effective End-of-Life Care." *Annals of Internal Medicine* 136, no. 9 (May 2002): 673–79.

Ersek, Mary, Marjorie Kawaga-Singer, Donelle Barnes, Leslie J. Blackhall, and Barbara A. Koenig. "Multicultural Considerations in the Use of Advance Directives." *Oncology Nursing Forum* 25, no. 10 (November–December 1998): 1683–90.

Galanti, Geri-Ann. *Caring For Patients from Different Cultures*. 3rd ed. Philadelphia: University of Pennsylvania Press, 2003.

Gaylin, Willard, and Bruce Jennings. *The Perversion of Autonomy: Coercion and Constraint in a Liberal Society*. Washington, D.C.: Georgetown University Press, 2003.

Green, Alexander R., Juan E. Carrillo, and Joseph R. Betancourt. "Why the Disease-Based Model of Medicine Fails Our Patients." *Western Journal of Medicine* 176, no. 2 (March 2002): 141–43.

Groce, Nora E., and Irving K. Zola. "Multiculturalism, Chronic Illness, and Disability." *Pediatrics* 91, no. 5 (May 1993): 1048–55. Cited in Martha O. Loustaunau and Elisa J. Sobo, *The Cultural Context of Health, Illness, and Medicine*. Westport, CT: Bergin & Garvey, 1997, 146.

Kagawa-Singer, Marjorie, and Shamsh Kassim-Lakha. "A Strategy to Reduce Cross-Cultural Miscommunication and Increase the Likelihood of Improving Health Outcomes." *Academic Medicine* 78, no. 6 (June 2003): 577–87.

Kleinman, Arthur, Leon Eisenberg, and Byron Good. "Culture, Illness, and Care: Clinical Lessons from Anthropologic and Cross-Cultural Research." *Annals of Internal Medicine* 88, no. 2 (February 1978): 251–58.

Koenig, Barbara A., and Jan Gates-Williams. "Understanding Cultural Difference in Caring for Dying Patients." *West Journal of Medicine* 163, no. 3 (September 1995): 244–49.

Kukoyi, Oladipo, Jason K. Wilbur, Mark A. Graber, and Hans House. "Case Studies in Cultural Competency." Pp. 389–404 in *Multicultural Medicine and Health Disparities*, edited by David Satcher and Rubens J. Pamies. New York: McGraw-Hill, 2005.

Loustaunau, Martha O., and Elisa J. Sobo. *The Cultural Context of Health, Illness, and Medicine*. Westport, CT: Bergin & Garvey, 1997.

Lynn, Joanne. "Why I Don't Have a Living Will." *Law, Medicine and Health Care* 19, no. 1–2 (Spring–Summer 1991):101–4.

Montgomery, Alan A., and Tom Fahey. "How Do Patients' Treatment Preferences Compare with Those of Clinicians?" *Quality in Health Care* 10, no. 1 (September 2001): i39–i43.

O'Neill, Onora. *Autonomy and Trust in Bioethics*. Cambridge, U.K.: Cambridge University Press, 2002.

Ripamonti, Carla. "International Perspectives: Italy." *Innovations in End-of-Life Care* 1, no. 1 (January–February 1999): 10. www2.edc.org/lastacts/archives/archivesjan99/intlpersp.asp#Italy (2003).

Searight, H. Russell, and Jennifer Gafford. "Cultural Diversity at the End of Life: Issues and Guidelines for Family Physicians." *American Family Physician* 71, no. 3 (February 2005): 515–22. www.aafp.org/afp/20050201/515.html (accessed March 12, 2009).

Swota, Alissa Hurwitz. "Cultural Diversity in the Clinical Setting." Pp. 107–32 in *Ethics By Committee*, edited by D. Micah Hester. Lanham, MD: Rowman & Littlefield Publishers, Inc., 2008.

Taylor, James S. "Autonomy and Informed Consent on the Navajo Reservation." *Journal of Social Philosophy* 35, no. 4 (Winter 2004): 506–16.

Turner, Leigh. "Bioethics and End-of-Life Care in Multi-Ethnic Settings: Cultural Diversity in Canada and the USA." *Mortality* 7, no. 3 (November 2002): 285–301.

——. "Bioethics in a Multicultural World: Medicine and Morality in Pluralistic Settings." *Health Care Analysis* 11, no. 2 (June 2003): 99–117.

Ulrich, Lawrence P. *The Patient Self-Determination Act: Meeting the Challenges in Patient Care*. Washington, D.C.: Georgetown University Press, 1999.

Werth Jr., James L., Dean Blevins, Karine L. Toussaint, and Martha R. Durham. "The Influence of Cultural Diversity on End-of-Life Care and Decisions." *American Behavioral Scientist* 46, no. 2 (October 2002): 204–19.

Wright, Fay, Shirlee Cohen, and Cynthia Caroselli. "Diverse Decisions. How Culture Affects Ethical Decision Making." *Critical Care Nursing Clinics of North America* 9, no. 1 (March 1997): 63–74.

Chapter One: Advance Care Planning: A Focus on Process

"Access & Diversity: Race and Ethnicity." *The University of British Columbia.* www.students.ubc.ca/access/race.cfm?page=glossary (accessed September 19, 2008).

"Advance Directives by State." *Wall Street Journal.* 2005. online.wsj.com/public/ article/SB111144394604885495-4MQpLbfZZSZWMXQ4BdPaL0 _1d0k_20050421.html?mod=tff_main_tff_top (accessed April 22, 2008).

Aging with Dignity. Five Wishes. www.agingwithdignity.org/5wishes.html.

Berry, Scott R., and Peter A. Singer. "The Cancer Specific Advance Directive." *Cancer* 82, no. 8 (April 1998): 1570–77.

Brody, Howard, and Timothy E. Quill. "Physician Recommendations and Patient Autonomy: Finding a Balance Between Physician Power and Patient Choice."*Annals of Internal Medicine* 125, no. 9 (November 1996): 763–69.

Browne, Alister, and Bill Sullivan. "Advance Directives in Canada." *Cambridge Quarterly of Healthcare Ethics* 15, no. 3 (Summer 2006): 256–60.

Canterbury v. Spence, 464 F.2d 772 (C.A.D.C. 1972).

Cantor, Norman L. "Prospective Autonomy: On the Limits of Shaping One's Post-Competence Medical Fate." *Journal of Contemporary Health Law and Policy* 8 (Spring 1992): 13–48.

——. *Advance Directives and the Pursuit of Death with Dignity.* Bloomington: Indiana University Press, 1993.

"Caring Conversations: Making your Wishes Known for End-of-Life Care." *Caring Conversations.* Center for Practical Bioethics. 2006. www.practicalbioethics. org/fileuploads/Caring%20Conversations.121406.pdf.

Chan, Ho Mun. "Sharing Death and Dying: Advance Directives, Autonomy, and the Family." *Bioethics* 18, no. 2 (April 2004): 87–103.

Christopher, Myra., ed. "Advance Care Planning—Part III: New Directions in Policy and Practice." *State Initiatives in End-of-Life Care* 23 (March 2005): 1–8. www. rwjf.org/files/publications/other/State_Initiatives_EOL23.pdf.

Cobbs v. Grant, 8 Cal. 3d 229, 502 P.2d 1 (1972).

Cotton, Paul. "Talk to People about Dying—They Can Handle it, Say Geriatricians and Patients." *Journal of the American Medical Association* 269, no. 3 (January 1993): 321–22.

Culver, Charles. "Advance Directives." *Psychology, Public Policy, and Law* 4, no. 3 (September 1998): 676–87.

Demons, Jamehl L., and Ramon Velez. "Geriatrics and End-of Life Care." Pp. 153–66 in *Multicultural Medicine and Health Disparities*, edited by David Satcher and Rubens J. Pamies. New York: McGraw-Hill, 2005.

DeSpelder, Lynne A., and Albert L. Strickland. *The Last Dance: Encountering Death and Dying.* New York: McGraw-Hill, 2001.

Ekblad, Solvig, Anneli Marttila, and Maria Emilsson. "Cultural Challenges in End-Of-Life Care: Reflections from Focus Groups' Interviews With Hospice Staff in Stockholm." *Journal of Advanced Nursing* 31, no. 3 (March 2000): 623–30.

Emanuel Linda L., and Ezekiel J. Emanuel. "The Medical Directive: A New Comprehensive Advance Care Document." *Journal of the American Medical Association* 261, no. 22 (June 1989): 3288–93.

Fagerlin, Angela, and Carl E. Schneider. "Enough: The Failure of the Living Will." *Hastings Center Report* 34, no. 2 (March–April 2004): 30–42.

Galanti, Geri-Ann. *Caring for Patients from Different Cultures.* 3rd ed. Philadelphia: University of Pennsylvania Press, 2004.

Hammes, Bernard, and Linda Briggs. "Respecting Choices: Key Components in Creating an Advance Care Planning Program." Gundersen Lutheran Medical Foundation, Inc. 2008. thehealthline.ca/Docs/RespectingChoices_Presentation.pdf.

Hilden, Hanna-Mari, Pekka Louhiala, and Jukka Palo. "End of Life Decisions: Attitudes of Finnish Physicians." *Journal of Medical Ethics* 30, no. 4 (2004): 362–65.

Kagawa-Singer, Marjorie, and Shamsh Kassim-Lakha. "A Strategy to Reduce Cross-Cultural Miscommunication and Increase the Likelihood of Improving Health Outcomes." *Academic Medicine* 78, no. 6 (June 2003): 577–87.

Katz, Jay. "Informed Consent—Must it Remain a Fairy Tale?" Pp. 92–100 in *Ethical Issues in Modern Medicine*, 6th ed., edited by Bonnie Steinbock, John D. Arras, and Alex John London. New York: McGraw-Hill, 2003.

Kettle, Nancy M. "Informed Consent in Clinical Practice." *Healthcare Ethics Committee Forum* 15, no. 1 (2003): 42–54.

Leahman, Dee. "Why the Patient Self-Determination Act Has Failed." *North Carolina Medical Journal* 65, no. 4 (July–August 2004): 249–51.

Lynn, Joanne. "Why I Don't Have a Living Will." *Law, Medicine and Health Care* 19, no. 1–2 (Spring–Summer 1991): 101–4.

Marshall, Patricia A., Barbara A. Koenig, Donelle Barnes, and Anne J. Davis. "Multiculturalism, Bioethics, and End-Of-Life Care: Case Narratives of Latino Cancer Patients." Pp. 421–31 in *Health Care Ethics: Critical Issues for the 21st Century*, edited by John F. Monagle and David C. Thomasma. Sudbury: Jones and Bartlett Publishers, 1998.

Murray, Thomas H., and Bruce Jennings. "The Quest to Reform End of Life Care: Rethinking Assumptions and Setting New Directions." *Hastings Center Report* 35, no. 6 supplement (November–December 2005): S52–57.

Natanson v. Kline, 186 Kan. 393, 350 P.2d 1093 (1960).

Natanson v. Kline, 187 Kan. 186, 354 P.2d 670 (1960).

Nuland, Sherwin B. *How We Die*. New York: Random House Inc., 1994.

O'Neill, Onora. *Autonomy and Trust in Bioethics*. Cambridge: Cambridge University Press, 2001.

Parker, Malcolm, Cameron Stewart, Lindy Willmott, and Colleen Cartwright. "Two Steps Forward, One Step Back: Advance Care Planning, Australian Regulatory Frameworks and the Australian Medical Association." *International Medicine Journal* 37, no. 9 (September 2007): 637–43.

Pearlman, Robert A., William G. Cole, Donald L. Patrick, Helene E. Starks, and Kevin C. Cain. "Advance Care Planning: Eliciting Patient Preferences for Life-Sustaining Treatment." *Patient Education and Counseling* 26, no. 1–3 (September 1995): 353–61.

Perkins, Henry S., Cynthia Geppert, Adelita Gonzalez, Josie D. Cortez, and Helen P. Hazuda. "Cross-Cultural Similarities and Differences in Attitudes about Advance

Care Planning." *Journal of General Internal Medicine* 17, no. 1 (January 2002): 48–57.

Quill, Timothy E. "Autonomy in a Relational Context: Balancing Individual, Family, Cultural, and Medical Interests." *Families, Systems & Health* 20, no. 3 (September 2002): 229–32.

Ripamonti, Carla. "International Perspectives: Italy." *Innovations in End-of-Life Care* 1, no. 1 (January–February 1999): 10. www2.edc.org/lastacts/archives/archivesjan99/intlpersp.asp#Italy (2003).

Rosenthal, Elizabeth. "Europeans are Grappling with Right-to-Die Issue: Living Wills Arrive, But Resistance Mounts." *International Herald Tribune*, May 16, 2007, page 1. www.ignaziomarino.it/Archivio/2/herald%20tribune.pdf (accessed April 8, 2009).

Salgo v. Leland Stanford Jr. University Bd. of Trustees, 154 Cal. App. 2d 560, 317 P.2d 170 (1957).

Schloendorff v. Society of New York Hospital, 211 N.Y. 125, 105 N.E. 92 (1914).

Shewchuk, Tara R. "Completing Advance Directives for Health Care Decisions: Getting to Yes." *Psychology, Public Policy, and Law* 4, no. 3 (September 1998): 703–18.

Singer, Peter A., Elaine C. Thiel, Irving Salit, William Flanagan, and Christopher D. Naylor. "The HIV-Specific Advance Directive." *Journal of General Internal Medicine* 12, no. 12 (December 1997): 729–35.

Swota, Alissa Hurwitz. "Cultural Diversity in the Clinical Setting." Pp. 107–132 in *Ethics By Committee*, edited by D. Micah Hester. Lanham, MD: Rowman & Littlefield Publishers, Inc., 2008.

Turner, Leigh. "Bioethics in a Multicultural World: Medicine and Morality in Pluralistic Settings." *Health Care Analysis* 11, no. 2 (June 2003): 99–117.

Ulrich, Lawrence P. *The Patient Self-Determination Act: Meeting the Challenges in Patient Care*. Washington, D.C.: Georgetown University Press, 1999.

van Oorschot, Birgill, and Alfred Simon. "Importance of the Advance Directive and the Beginning of the Dying Process from the Point of View of German Doctors and Judges Dealing with Guardianship Matters: Results of an Empirical Survey." *Journal of Medical Ethics* 32, no. 11 (November 2006): 623–26.

Voltz, Raymond, Akira Akabayashi, Carol Reese, Gen Ohi, and Hans-Martin Sass. "End-of-Life Decisions and Advance Directives in Palliative Care: A Cross-Cultural Survey of Patients and Health-Care Professionals." *Journal of Pain and Symptom Management* 16, no. 3 (September 1998): 153–62.

Waters, Catherine M. "Understanding and Supporting African Americans' Perspectives of End-of-Life Care Planning and Decision Making." *Qualitative Health Research* 11, no. 3 (May 2001): 385–98.

Webb, Marilyn. *The Good Death: The New American Search to Reshape the End of Life*. New York: Bantam Books, 1999.

Zimring, Stuart D. "Multi-Cultural Issues in Advance Directives." *Journal of the American Medical Directors Association* 2, no. 5 (September–October 2001): 241–45.

Zylicz, Zbigniew. "International Perspectives: The Netherlands." *Innovations In End-of-Life Care* 1, no. 1 (January–February 1999): 12. www2.edc.org/lastacts/archives/archivesJan99/intlpersp.asp#The%20Netherlands (2003).

Chapter Two: A Plurality of Cultures

Bronheim, Suzanne, and Suganya Sockalingam. "A Guide to Choosing and Adapting Culturally and Linguistically Competent Health Promotion Materials." *National Center for Cultural Competence* (Winter/Spring 2003): 1–12.

Fadiman, Anne. *The Spirit Catches You and You Fall Down*. New York: Farrar, Straus and Giroux, 1998.

Frederick, Robert E. "An Outline of Ethical Relativism and Ethical Absolutism." Pp. 65–80 in *A Companion to Business Ethics*, edited by Robert E. Frederick. Oxford, U.K.: Blackwell Publishers Ltd., 1999.

Galanti, Geri-Ann. *Caring for Patients from Different Cultures*. 3rd ed. Philadelphia: University of Pennsylvania Press, 2004.

Internet Encyclopedia of Philosophy, s.v. "Human Rights." www.iep.utm.edu/h/humrts.htm#SH5a.

Jennings, Bruce. "Values Near the End of Lives: Grassroots Perspectives and Cultural Diversity on End-of-Life Care." American Health Decisions (position papers) (May 1999). www.ahd.org/Values_Near_the_End_of_Lives.html (accessed April 22, 2009).

Kagawa-Singer, Marjorie, and Shamsh Kassim-Lakha. "A Strategy to Reduce Cross-Cultural Miscommunication and Increase the Likelihood of Improving Health Outcomes." *Academic Medicine* 78, no. 6 (June 2003): 577–87.

Koenig, Barbara A., and Jan Gates-Williams. "Understanding Cultural Difference in Caring for Dying Patients." *West Journal of Medicine* 163, no. 3: (September 1995): 244–49.

Krakauer, Eric L., Chris Crenner, and Ken Fox. "Barriers to Optimum End-of-Life Care for Minority Patients." *Journal of the American Geriatrics Society* 50, no. 1 (January 2002): 182–90. Cited in James L. Werth Jr., Dean Blevins, Karine L. Toussaint, and Martha R. Durham, "The Influence of Cultural Diversity on End-of-Life Care and Decisions," *American Behavioral Scientist* 46, no. 2 (October 2002): 204–19.

Lewis, Toby. "Somali Cultural Profile." *EthnoMed*. University of Washington and the Harborview Medical Center. 1996. ethnomed.org/ethnomed/cultures/somali/somali_cp.html (accessed June 20, 2007).

Loustaunau, Martha O., and Elisa J. Sobo. *The Cultural Context of Health, Illness, and Medicine*. Westport, CT: Bergin & Garvey, 1997.

Macklin, Ruth. "Ethical Relativism in a Multicultural Society." *Kennedy Institute of Ethics Journal* 8, no. 1 (March 1998): 1–22.

——. *Against Relativism: Cultural Diversity and the Search for Ethical Universals in Medicine*. Oxford, New York: Oxford University Press, 1999.

Merriam-Webster Online Dictionary, s.v. "health."

——, s.v. "illness."

Mulhall, Anne. "The Cultural Context of Death: What Nurses Need to Know." *Nursing Times* 92, no. 34 (August 1996): 38–40.

Orr, Robert D. "Treating Patients from Other Cultures." *American Family Physician* 53, no. 6 (May 1996): 2004–6.

Perkins, Henry S., Cynthia Geppert, Adelita Gonzalez, Josie D. Cortez, and Helen P. Hazuda. "Cross-Cultural Similarities and Differences in Attitudes about Advance Care Planning." *Journal of General Internal Medicine* 17, no. 1 (January 2002): 48–57.

Rachels, James, and Stuart Rachels. *The Elements of Moral Philosophy*. 5th ed. New York: McGraw-Hill, 2006.

Spector, Rachel E. *Cultural Diversity in Health and Illness*. 6th ed. Upper Saddle River, NJ: Prentice Hall, 2003.

Swota, Alissa Hurwitz. "Cultural Diversity in the Clinical Setting." Pp. 107–132 in *Ethics By Committee*, edited by D. Micah Hester. Lanham, MD: Rowman & Littlefield Publishers, Inc., 2008.

Timmons, Mark. *Moral Theory: An Introduction*. Lanham, MD: Rowman & Littlefield Publishers, Inc., 2002.

Turner, Leigh. "Bioethics and End-of-Life Care in Multi-Ethnic Settings: Cultural Diversity in Canada and the USA." *Mortality* 7, no. 3 (2002): 285–301.

———. "Bioethics in a Multicultural World: Medicine and Morality in Pluralistic Settings." *Health Care Analysis* 11, no. 2 (June 2003): 99–117.

"What's Culture Got To Do With It? Excising the Harmful Tradition of Female Circumcision." *Harvard Law Review* 106, no. 8 (June 1993): 1944–61.

Chapter Three: Communication Across Cultures

Andrulis, Dennis, Nanette Goodman, and Carol Pryor. "What a Difference an Interpreter Can Make: Health Care Experiences of Uninsured with Limited English Proficiency." The Access Project. 2002. www.accessproject.org/downloads/c_LEP-Engembarg.pdf (accessed August 22, 2007).

Boyles, Salynn. "Language Barrier Affecting Health Care: Proper Medical Care May Be Hampered by Lack of Qualified Interpreters." *WebMD Health News*. 2006. www.webmd.com/news/20060719/language-barrier-affecting-health-care.

Chesanow, Neil. "The Versatile Doctor's Guide to Ethnic Diversity." *Medical Economics* 75, no. 17 (September 1998): 135–46.

Crawley, LaVera M., Patricia A. Marshall, Bernard Lo, and Barbara A. Koenig. "Strategies for Culturally Effective End-of-Life Care." *Annals of Internal Medicine* 136, no. 9 (May 2002): 673–79.

"Cultural Competence Works: Using Cultural Competence to Improve the Quality of Health Care for Diverse Populations and Add Value to Managed Care Arrangements." Health Resources and Services Administration. 2001. ftp.hrsa.gov/financeMC/cultural-competence.pdf.

Flores, Glenn. "Culture and the Patient-Physician Relationship: Achieving Cultural Competency in Health Care." *Journal of Pediatrics* 136, no. 1 (January 2000): 14–23.

Flores, Glenn, Michael B. Laws, Sandra J. Mayo, Barry Zuckerman, Milagros Abreu, Leonardo Medina, and Eric J. Hardt. "Errors in Medical Interpretation and Their Potential Consequences in Pediatric Encounters." *Pediatrics* 111, no. 1 (January 2003): 6–14.

Galanti, Geri-Ann. *Caring for Patients from Different Cultures*. 3rd ed. Philadelphia: University of Pennsylvania Press, 2004.

Groce, Nora E., and Irving K. Zola. "Multiculturalism, Chronic Illness, and Disability." *Pediatrics* 91, no. 5 (May 1993): 1048–55. Cited in Martha O. Loustaunau and Elisa J. Sobo, *The Cultural Context of Health, Illness, and Medicine* (Westport, CT: Bergin & Garvey, 1997), 146.

Hallenbeck, James, Mary K. Goldstein, and Eric W. Mebane. "Cultural Considerations of Death and Dying in the United States." *Clinics in Geriatric Medicine* 12, no. 2 (May 1996): 393–406.

Hudelson, Patricia. "Improving Patient—Provider Communication: Insights from Interpreters." *Family Practice* 22, no. 3 (June 2005): 311–16.

Jennings, Bruce. "Values Near the End of Lives: Grassroots Perspectives and Cultural Diversity on End-of-Life Care." American Health Decisions (position papers) (May 1999). www.ahd.org/Values_Near_the_End_of_Lives.html (accessed April 22, 2009).

Kagawa-Singer, Marjorie, and Shamsh Kassim-Lakha. "A Strategy to Reduce Cross-Cultural Miscommunication and Increase the Likelihood of Improving Health Outcomes." *Academic Medicine* 78, no. 6 (June 2003): 577–87.

Orona, Celia J., Barbara A. Koenig, and Anne J. Davis. "Cultural Aspects of Nondisclosure." *Cambridge Quarterly of Healthcare Ethics* 3, no. 3 (Summer 1994): 338–46.

Quill, Timothy E. "Autonomy in a Relational Context: Balancing Individual, Family, Cultural, and Medical Interests." *Families, Systems & Health* 20, no. 3 (September 2002): 229–32.

Shaw, George B. Quoted in James Hallenbeck, Mary K. Goldstein, and Eric W. Mebane, "Cultural Considerations of Death and Dying in the United States." *Clinics in Geriatric Medicine* 12, no. 2 (May 1996): 397.

Trotter, Robert T. "National Health Service Corps Educational Program for Clinical and Community Issues in Primary Care: Cross-Cultural Issues in Primary Care Module." American Medical Student Association/Foundation. www.amsa.org/pdf/culture.pdf (accessed July 16, 2008).

U.S. Department of Health and Human Services. "National Standards for Culturally and Linguistically Appropriate Services in Health Care: Final Report." The Office of Minority Health. 2001. www.omhrc.gov/assets/pdf/checked/finalreport.pdf (accessed December 2008).

Welch, Melissa. "Care of Blacks and African Americans." Pp. 29–60 in *Cross-Cultural Medicine*, edited by Judyann Bigby. Philadelphia: American College of Physicians, 2001.

Chapter Four: Truth-Telling and Disclosure

Aging with Dignity. Five Wishes. www.agingwithdignity.org/5wishes.html.

Arras, John D., and Bonnie Steinbock, eds. *Ethical Issues in Modern Medicine*. 5th ed. New York: McGraw-Hill, 1998.

Beyene, Yewoubdar. "Medical Disclosure and Refugees. Telling Bad News to Ethiopian Patients." *The Western Journal of Medicine* 157, no. 3 (September 1992): 328–32.

Bito, Seiji, Shinji Matsumura, Marjorie Kawaga-Singer, Lisa S. Meredith, Shinichi Fukuhara, and Neil S. Wenger. "Acculturation and End-of-Life Decision Making: Comparison of Japanese and Japanese-American Focus Groups." *Bioethics* 21, no. 5 (June 2007): 251–62.

Brotzman, Gregory L., and Dennis J. Butler. "Cross-Cultural Issues in the Disclosure of a Terminal Diagnosis: A Case Report." *The Journal of Family Practice* 32, no. 4 (April 1991): 426–27.

Candib, Lucy M. *Medicine and the Family: A Feminist Perspective.* New York: Basic Books, 1995.

——. "Truth Telling and Advance Planning at the End of Life: Problems with Autonomy in a Multicultural World." *Families, Systems, and Health* 20, no. 3 (September 2002): 213–28.

Chan, Ho Mun. "Sharing Death and Dying: Advance Directives, Autonomy, and the Family." *Bioethics* 18, no. 2 (April 2004): 87–103.

Emanuel Linda L., and Ezekiel J. Emanuel. "The Medical Directive: A New Comprehensive Advance Care Document." *Journal of the American Medical Association* 261, no. 22 (June 1989): 3288–93.

Fan, Ruiping. "Self-Determination vs. Family-Determination: Two Incommensurable Principles of Autonomy." *Bioethics* 11, no. 3–4 (July–October 1997): 309–22.

Gordon, Deborah R., and Eugenio Paci. "Disclosure Practices and Cultural Narratives: Understanding Concealment and Silence Around Cancer in Tuscany, Italy." *Social Science and Medicine* 44, no. 10 (May 1997): 1433–52.

Gostin, Lawrence O. "Informed Consent, Cultural Sensitivity, and Respect for Persons." *Journal of the American Medical Association* 274, no. 10 (September 1995): 844–45.

Hudelson, Patricia. "Improving Patient—Provider Communication: Insights from Interpreters." *Family Practice* 22, no. 3 (June 2005): 311–16.

Kagawa-Singer, Marjorie, and Shamsh Kassim-Lakha. "A Strategy to Reduce Cross-Cultural Miscommunication and Increase the Likelihood of Improving Health Outcomes." *Academic Medicine* 78, no. 6 (June 2003): 577–87.

Kimura, Rihito. "Death, Dying, and Advance Directives in Japan: Socio-Cultural and Legal Point of View." *Advance Directive and Surrogate Decision Making in Transcultural Perspective.* Baltimore: Johns Hopkins University Press, 1998.

MacDonald, Neil. *Palliative Medicine: A Case-Based Manual.* Oxford, England: Oxford University Press, 1998.

Orona, Celia J., Barbara A. Koenig, and Anne J. Davis. "Cultural Aspects of Nondisclosure." *Cambridge Quarterly of Healthcare Ethics* 3, no. 3 (Summer 1994): 338–46.

Orr, Robert D. "Treating Patients from Other Cultures." *American Family Physician* 53, no. 6 (May 1996): 2004–6.

Parry, Joan K., and Angela S. Ryan. *A Cross-Cultural Look at Death, Dying, and Religion.* Chicago: Nelson-Hall, 1995.

Werth Jr., James L., Dean Blevins, Karine L. Toussaint, and Martha R. Durham. "The Influence of Cultural Diversity on End-of-Life Care and Decisions." *American Behavioral Scientist* 46, no. 2 (October 2002): 204–19.

Zimring, Stuart D. "Multi-Cultural Issues in Advance Directives." *Journal of the American Medical Directors Association* 2, no. 5 (September–October 2001): 241–45.

Chapter Five: Realizing the Goal of Cultural Sensitivity in the Clinical Setting—Where the Rubber Hits the Road

Berlin, Elois Ann, and William C. Fowkes, Jr. "Cross-Cultural Medicine: A Teaching Framework for Cross-Cultural Health Care—Application in Family Practice." *The Western Journal of Medicine* 139, no. 6 (1983): 934–38.

Bronheim, Suzanne, and Suganya Sockalingam. "A Guide to Choosing and Adapting Culturally and Linguistically Competent Health Promotion Materials." *National Center for Cultural Competence* (Winter–Spring 2003): 1–12.

Butterfield, Stacey. "A Different Kind of Competency: Growing Immigrant Population Spurs New Regulations, Education Programs." *ACP Hospitalist.* 2008. www.acponline.org/ clinical_information/journals_publications/acp_hospitalist/mar08/cover.htm (accessed July 16, 2008).

Chan, Ho Mun. "Sharing Death and Dying: Advance Directives, Autonomy, and the Family." *Bioethics* 18, no. 2 (April 2004): 87–103.

Crandall, Sonia J., Geeta George, Gail S. Marion, and Steve Davis. "Applying Theory to the Design of Cultural Competency Training for Medical Students: A Case Study." *Academic Medicine* 78, no. 6 (June 2003): 588–94.

"Cultural Competency Laws." *American College of Physicians.* 2005. www.acponline.org/ advocacy/state_policy/reports/10-28-05.pdf (accessed July 16, 2008).

Ersek, Mary, Marjorie Kawaga-Singer, Donelle Barnes, Leslie J. Blackhall, and Barbara A. Koenig. "Multicultural Considerations in the Use of Advance Directives." *Oncology Nursing Forum* 25, no. 10 (November–December 1998): 1683–90.

"Ethnicity and Cancer Patient Information: Key Learning Points from the Literature Review of the NCA's 2nd Phase." *National Cancer Alliance.* 2001. www.teamworkfile.org.uk/download/TW2%20S%20Asian%20Lit%20Review.pdf. Cited in Kyriaki Mystakidou, Eleni Tsilika, Efi Parpa, Emmanuela Katsouda, and Lambros Vlahos, "Patterns and Barriers in Information Disclosure between Health Care Professionals and Relatives with Cancer Patients in Greek Society." *European Journal of Cancer Care* 14, no. 2 (May 2005): 175–81.

Flores, Glenn. "Culture and the Patient-Physician Relationship: Achieving Cultural Competency in Health Care." *Journal of Pediatrics* 136, no. 1 (January 2000): 14–23.

Freedman, Benjamin. "Offering Truth: One Ethical Approach to the Uninformed Cancer Patient." Pp. 110–16 in *Ethical Issues in Modern Medicine*, 7th ed., edited by Bonnie Steinbock, John D. Arras, and Alex J. London. New York: McGraw-Hill, 2008.

Fryer-Edwards Kelly, Robert Arnold, Anthony Back, Walter Baile, and James Tulsky "Fundamentals of Communication." In *Tough Talk: Helping Doctors Approach Difficult Conversations.* Available at: depts.washington.edu/toolbox/.

———. "Module 1: Fundamental Communication Skills." *Medical Oncology Communication Skills Learning Modules.* 2002. depts.washington.edu/oncotalk/learn/modules/Modules_01.pdf.

———. "Module 4: Talking about Advance Care Plans and Do Not Resuscitate Orders." *Medical Oncology Communication Skills Learning Modules.* 2002. depts.washington.edu/oncotalk/learn/modules/Modules_04.pdf.

Gandhi, Mohandas. thinkexist.com/quotation/i_do_not_want_my_house_to_be_walled_in_on_all/10833.html (accessed July 2008).

Giger, Joyce N., and Ruth Davidhizar. "The Giger and Davidhizar Transcultural Assessment Model." *Journal of Transcultural Nursing* 13, no. 3 (July 2002): 185–88.

Giger, Joyce N., Ruth Davidhizar, and Pamela Fordham. "Multi-Cultural and Multi-Ethnic Considerations and Advance Directives: Developing Cultural Competency." *Journal of Cultural Diversity* 13, no. 1 (Spring 2006): 3–9.

"A Guide to Infusing Cultural & Linguistic Competence in Health Promotion Training: Group Activity—Understanding the Cultural Competence Continuum." National Center for Cultural Competence. www11.georgetown.edu/research/gucchd/nccc/projects/sids/dvd/continuum.pdf (accessed November 2006).

"A Guide to Infusing Cultural & Linguistic Competence in Health Promotion Training: Group Activity—Who Lives in Our Area." National Center for Cultural Competence. www11.georgetown.edu/research/gucchd/NCCC/projects/sids/dvd/demographics.pdf.

Hallenbeck, James, and Mary K. Goldstein. "Decisions at the End of Life: Cultural Considerations Beyond Medical Ethics." *Generations* 23, no. 1 (Spring 1999): 24–29.

James, Erin. "Ethno-Experts: When Researching Cultures, Learn the Most from Your Community Resources." *Advance for Nurses* 7, no. 14 (2005): 25–26. nursing.advanceweb.com/Editorial/Content/Editorial.aspx?CC=133164 (accessed April 9, 2009).

The Joint Commission. *About The Joint Commission.* 2008. www.jointcommission.org/AboutUs/ (accessed July 17, 2008).

"The Joint Commission 2008 Requirements Related to the Provision of Culturally and Linguistically Appropriate Health Care: April 2008." The Joint Commission. 2008. www.jointcommission.org/NR/rdonlyres/6941959E-D4BE-48D7-A2F8-A4834E84B263/0/JC_Standards_Document_2008.pdf (accessed January 27, 2009).

Kagawa-Singer, Marjorie, and Leslie Blackhall. "Negotiating Cross-Cultural Issues at the End of Life." *Journal of the American Medical Association*, 286 (2001): 2993–3001.

Kleinman, Arthur. *Patients and Healers in the Context of Culture.* Berkeley: University of California Press, 1981.

Kleinman, Arthur, Leon Eisenberg, and Byron Good. "Culture, Illness, and Care: Clinical Lessons from Anthropologic and Cross-Cultural Research." *Annals of Internal Medicine* 88, no. 2 (February 1978): 251–58.

Koenig, Barbara A. "Cultural Diversity in Decisionmaking about Care at the End of Life." Pp. 363–82 in *Approaching Death: Improving Care at the End-of-Life*, edited by Marilyn J. Field and Christine K. Cassel. Washington, D.C.: National Academy Press, 1997.

Koenig Barbara A., and Jan Gates-Williams. "Understanding Cultural Difference in Caring for Dying Patients." *West Journal of Medicine* 163, no. 3 (September 1995): 244–49.

Leininger, Madeleine M., and Marilyn R. McFarland. *Culture Care Diversity and Universality: A Worldwide Nursing Theory*. 2nd ed. Sudbury, MA: Jones and Bartlett, 2006.

Mead, Margaret. www.diversityatwork.com.au/node/1017 (July 2008).

Migration Information Source. Migration Policy Institute. 2009. www.migrationin-formation.org/

National Center for Health Statistics. Centers for Disease Control and Prevention. 2009. www.cdc.gov/nchs/Default.htm.

National Standards on Culturally and Linguistically Appropriate Service. Office of Minority Health. 2007. www.omhrc.gov/templates/browse.aspx?lvl=2&lvlid=15 (accessed January 21, 2009).

Parry, Joan K., and Angela S. Ryan. *A Cross-Cultural Look at Death, Dying, and Religion*. Chicago: Nelson-Hall, 1995.

Quill, Timothy E. "Autonomy in a Relational Context: Balancing Individual, Family, Cultural, and Medical Interests." *Families, Systems & Health* 20, no. 3 (September 2002): 229–32.

Searight, H. Russell, and Jennifer Gafford. "Cultural Diversity at the End of Life: Issues and Guidelines for Family Physicians." *American Family Physician* 71, no. 3 (February 2005): 515–22. www.aafp.org/afp/20050201/515.html (accessed March 12, 2009).

Smedley, Brian D., Adrienne Y. Stith, and Alan R. Nelson., eds. "Interventions: Cross-Cultural Education in the Health Professions." Pp. 199–214 in *Unequal Treatment: Confronting Racial and Ethnic Disparities in Health Care*. 2003. www.nap.edu/openbook.php?isbn=030908265X&page=199.

Spector, Rachel E. *Cultural Diversity in Health and Illness*. 6th ed. Upper Saddle River, NJ: Prentice Hall, 2003.

Taylor, Andrew, and Margaret Box. "Multicultural Palliative Care Guidelines." Palliative Care Australia. 1999. www.palliativecare.org.au/Portals/46/resources/MulticulturalGuidelines.pdf.

Taylor, David, and Peter A. Cameron. "Advance Care Planning in Australia: Overdue for Improvement." *Internal Medicine Journal* 32, no. 9–10 (September–October 2002): 475–80.

Voltz, Raymond, Akira Akabayashi, Carol Reese, Gen Ohi, and Hans-Martin Sass. "End-of-Life Decisions and Advance Directives in Palliative Care: A Cross-Cultural Survey of Patients and Health-Care Professionals." *Journal of Pain and Symptom Management* 16, no. 3 (September 1998): 153–62.

Werth Jr., James L., Dean Blevins, Karine L. Toussaint, and Martha R. Durham. "The Influence of Cultural Diversity on End-of-Life Care and Decisions." *American Behavioral Scientist* 46, no. 2 (October 2002): 204–19.

Wright, Fay, Shirlee Cohen, and Cynthia Caroselli. "Diverse Decisions. How Culture Affects Ethical Decision Making." *Critical Care Nursing Clinics of North America* 9, no. 1 (March 1997): 63–74.

Index

About the Author

Alissa Hurwitz Swota, PhD, is an assistant professor of philosophy at the University of North Florida and senior fellow in bioethics at the Blue Cross Blue Shield of Northeast Florida Center for Ethics, Public Policy, and the Professions. She is also clinical bioethicist at Wolfson Children's Hospital in Jacksonville, Florida. She received her PhD in philosophy with a concentration in medical ethics at the University at Albany State University of New York, and completed a postdoctoral fellowship in clinical ethics at the University of Toronto Joint Centre for Bioethics. She has published in professional journals and has authored chapters in books on clinical ethics consultation and educating members of hospital ethics committees. Her research focuses on decision-making at the end of life, cultural issues in the clinical setting, pediatric bioethics, and advance care planning.

Lightning Source UK Ltd.
Milton Keynes UK
UKHW041828120722
405770UK00001B/12